MADE FOR LAUGHTER

MADE FOR
LAUGHTER

Sheila Cassidy

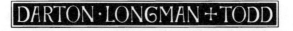
DARTON·LONGMAN+TODD

First published in 2006 by
Darton, Longman and Todd Ltd
1 Spencer Court
140–142 Wandsworth High Street
London SW18 4JJ

ISBN 0 232 52248 0

A catalogue record for this book is available from the British Library.

Designed and produced by Sandie Boccacci
Phototypeset in 10.75/13.5pt Minion
Printed and bound in Great Britain by
Page Bros, Norwich, Norfolk

*To all those friends and family
who make my life so rich and happy, especially
John Garner, Carole Evans, Jacky Clift and Martin Sellix*

'We are made for goodness, we are made for love, we are made for laughter, we are made for joy, we are made for transcendence.'

Desmond Tutu

CONTENTS

ACKNOWLEDGEMENTS

My thanks are due to all who have worked with me to bring this book to birth: Clare and Anne Hallward and Neil McKenty who read the early chapters and shamed me into total honesty; Rosalie Shaw, who worried about my being too honest; Carole Evans, who took pity on my cyber-phobia and typed the initial chapters, and Pam Gelhouse who patiently typed and retyped the whole manuscript; Martin Sellix, who read and commented on the work in progress; Sophie Stanes for providing the front cover photograph, and lastly Brendan Walsh, my genial editor, who sustained me with chocolate and helpful comment during the long months of writing.

SHEILA CASSIDY
Plymouth 2006

1

EARLY DAYS

This is the story of the journey undertaken by one rather idiosyncratic woman, her friends, relations, dogs and other animals. It begins in Lincolnshire two years before the outbreak of the Second World War and takes us up to time of writing in Plymouth in 2006. It is an unashamedly Roman Catholic story of a convent schoolgirl, tormented by thoughts of becoming a nun for over twenty years, until she entered a convent at the age of forty only to be thrown out eighteen months later because she was so miserable. In fact, being thrown out of places forms a recurring theme, including expulsion from Chile by the secret police and dismissal from a hospice for the dying for accepting too many lecture engagements. Enough: let me begin.

I am what is sometimes called a cradle Catholic: born to Catholic parents and educated by nuns. Now although technically lapsed, in that I no longer feel obliged to go to Mass on Sunday, I still count myself a Catholic, for as the disciples said to Jesus, 'Lord, to whom shall we go?' By this I mean that I have no inclination to become an Anglican, a Buddhist, a Muslim or even a Quaker because I find institutionalised religion too confining and, for the moment, I prefer to live my life without it. Perhaps, before I die, I shall come back to the Church, as Catholics are prone to do, but if that happens it will be for my need, not God's. By this I mean that it is *we*, who at various times of our lives, need to worship with other people and in a formal way. God does not 'need' us to do that. He or She does not 'need' our worship though I believe God 'needs' our love. (Please don't ask me what I mean by the statement that God needs our love: I know it in my guts, not in my head!)

Although I no longer go to church I still pray, briefly and formally in the early morning as I drink my tea, as well as off and on a good deal during the day. A lot of my prayer these days is without words: odd movements of the heart in response to the beauty of nature or the constant delight afforded me by my dogs. I pray that God be in my head as I teach at the hospice and in my understanding as I sit listening to my psychotherapy clients. I pray too, quite shamelessly, for God to find me a parking place as I approach my home and am amazed that it always seems to work.

I pray only occasionally for the suffering world: the sick, the dying and the refugees. My intuition tells me that God has this in hand: what manner of a God would withhold healing or peace because not enough people have asked for it? I believe that God is irretrievably caught up in the joy and the pain of the world, living, laughing, crying and dying in and with us all the world over.

So, how did I arrive at this place of belief and belonging? As I said earlier, I am a cradle Catholic, born to a Catholic father and a mother who converted when she married him. Ours was not the archetypal Anglo-Irish Catholic home with pictures of the Sacred Heart, statues of the Virgin and nightly family rosary: far from it. My father's was a punctilious and somewhat rigid observance and my mother's an openly resentful one. Frankly, she hated Catholicism in general and the Pope in particular, largely, I think, because of the birth-control issue. I was an accidental and belated product of their union and I suspect it took her a while to come to terms with the idea of another baby and a girl at that.

My mother, born Barbara Margaret Drew, was a widely read, artistic woman, good with her hands and with colour, who had a passion for animals. She was the eldest of five children born to Harvey Richard Drew, one of the founders of the London Stockbrokers Philips and Drew. Her mother was Margery Ashworth, a gentle and kindly woman whose parents had come from Lancashire and the cotton mills. Although I spent several months with my grandparents in the early days of the 1939–45 war, I have few memories of them, though their house 'Milburn Orchard' overlooking a Devon estuary came to symbolise for me all that was good and beautiful about life and summer holidays.

Milburn was built during the 1920s as a holiday home for the Drews: my mother, her brothers Humphrey, David and Edmund and her equally artistic and eccentric sister Anne. During the rest of the year they lived in Surrey. When the Second World War broke out the boys joined the forces, Humphrey becoming a gunner, David a naval officer and Edmund a pilot in the Royal Air Force. My mother, meanwhile, lived at home, working briefly as a postwoman and pursuing her art. History has it that she was very beautiful and had many suitors but had eyes for none of them after she met my father, a charismatic Australian officer in the newly formed Royal Air Force.

My father, born in Queensland in 1890, was a man of powerful intellect and personality. He had bushy eyebrows and piercing blue eyes and, as a small girl I adored him. He was a child of the Australian out-back, son of Northern Irish immigrants, Faris Cassidy and Jane Callaghan from County Fermanagh who had left Ireland after the famine, around 1850. Faris became manager of a large sheep station and my father rode his pony to school each day. His secondary schooling was at Nudgee, a big Catholic school in Brisbane run by the Irish Christian brothers. He went on to become a foundation student at the new University of Queensland and was awarded a Rhodes Scholarship to Oxford University in 1913 where he proposed to study 'scientific agri-culture' and was, I think, thought of as a candidate for the Chair of Agriculture at the University of Queensland.

The war, however, changed his life, for he joined the army and served in Gallipoli, clearly with some distinction as he was awarded the DSO (Distinguished Service Order). After the war, he returned to Oxford as an officer and eventually transferred to the Royal Air Force.

By the time the Second World War broke out in 1939 I was two and my parents were living in Lincolnshire at Cranwell, the Royal Air Force College where my father was senior lecturer in the Electrical Wireless School. He was immediately posted to Stanmore where he was Chief Signals Officer at Fighter Command. My mother and my brother Mike, then eight years old, went with him while my sister Margaret, aged fifteen, returned to her French convent school, Les Oiseaux, where, she told me, they were instructed that it was a mortal sin to sit on the grass! I, the baby of the family at just two years old, was 'evacuated' to my grandparents who were by then living permanently in Devon. I'm sure these arrange-ments were made in good faith, but in hindsight, the move must have been a very damaging one for me.

At Cranwell I had been cared for by a very loving nanny, but when I was sent away she could not accompany me so I was put in the care of Ellen, a local sixteen-year-old girl. Poor Ellen: how she must have hated Milburn and its inhabitants! The house is built on a steep hillside overlooking the estuary; the nearest village, Aveton Gifford, is about three-quarters of a mile away. The road crosses the river at right angles and then runs parallel with it, and is covered twice a day by the tide. This, of course, is why my grandparents loved it, for Drews are loners, protective of their privacy and needing no company other than family members and their animals, but poor Ellen must have experienced it as a prison.

Ellen and I were thrown together with only Violet, the rather taciturn cook, for company. Each day at four I was presented to my grandparents as they took their afternoon tea and allowed to play briefly with the toys from the special toy cupboard in the drawing room. The rest of the day would have been spent in the servants' sitting room, adjacent to the kitchen, which my Uncle Humphrey much later converted into a stable for his horse Fred.

The garden was not in the least child friendly, steep at the back and terraced at the front in massive six-foot steps. For an older child it would have been idyllic, with endless places to hide and play, but for a two-year-old it can only have been out of bounds. Inside the house was no better: my grandparents' rooms were on the first floor, but I'm not sure where I slept. It must been in the spare room or else up in the attic, which was accessed by a steep, almost vertical, staircase. In either situation I must have been locked in for safety, lest I break my neck falling down the stairs.

I have thought a lot about this time over the years but have been unable to remember people or events. All I can do is imagine myself into my two-year-old self and the minds of my keepers, and my guess is that I was a very lonely and unhappy little girl cared for by an even more lonely and frustrated teenager. Ellen would likely have been completely isolated from people of her own age because any outing would have been on foot and seriously limited by fear of being cut off by the tide.

Ironically, this incarceration could be understood as the 'secret' of my later success. Unable to understand why my parents had 'rejected' me by sending me away, I tried ever harder to please the grown-ups in the hope that I might be restored to my family, especially my brother Mike whom I adored all my childhood. Just how long I spent in Devon no one left alive can remember. My brother was a weekly boarder at school and my sister was trying to escape the watchful eye of the nuns, while I sat sadly on the stairs at Milburn, watching and waiting for someone to come and take me home.

Around 1941 or 1942 my father was named Air Officer Commanding No. 27 Group and we moved to live at the Royal Agricultural College, just outside Cirencester, which had been taken over by the Air Force. By now I was four or five years old and very much happier in the care of a delightful Scottish nanny called Elsie, a WAAF under my father's command. My mother as usual was busy with her embroidery and two cairn terriers while my father was endlessly occupied by his work as a leader of men.

John Reginald Cassidy (known all my life as Michael) was a man used to command, but he was also very loving of his family, especially of my mother and myself. I was his blue-eyed baby girl and my earliest memories are of riding high on his shoulders, feeling like a princess. He used to read to Mike and me and I remember sitting in the double bed listening enchanted as he read *Robinson Crusoe* and *Treasure Island*.

There was, however, another side to my father, which marred the very close relationship between us. He was extremely proud of me but also very demanding, so that in later years I felt possessed by his love in a way which became increasingly uncomfortable. There was also a single episode in which he beat me for letting him down: I had been rude to some important visitors and, when they had left, he woke me from sleep to chastise me with his bare hand. It sounds such a little thing: a one-off spanking which I should have long since forgotten. The fact is, however, that I have very clear memories of the event which felt like a betrayal by both parents: my father for beating me and my mother for not stopping him.

When I was old enough, I was taken to Sunday Mass with my father and brother while my mother stayed behind to cook the Sunday lunch. One day, when I was quite small, I forgot to take my much-hated school hat and when my father realised I was hatless he refused to allow me to accompany him into the church. After all, he *was* the Air Commodore (or was it the Air Vice-Marshal) and had to keep up appearances! That day I learned my first piece of intuitive or God-given theology – God does not give a fig about hats in church. As I sat in the back of the official car, with the chauffeur no doubt having a fag nearby, I knew that God loved me with or without my hat and that he was there in the car with me as well as (or perhaps instead of) in the church. In later years I used to test these theories by calling upon God in his sundry houses clad in whatever I happened to be wearing: normally shorts and a shirt. I decided around that time (my early teens) that I would like to go to Mass every day *except* on Sundays. I think what I really liked about weekday Mass was that there weren't many takers whereas on Sundays all the world and his wife were there and I felt crowded and uncomfortable.

Mine was a Second World War childhood and we lived in considerable style in the Principal's house at the College. When I was seven or eight, however, I developed asthma and the GP, for reasons best known to himself, advised that I should go to boarding school, and I was consigned therefore to the local convent. Most of the nuns were, I think, German – and of course we were at war with Germany. My memories are not really happy ones; I was homesick but I was not maltreated in any way. (How awful to have to say that, but knowing as I do that many Catholic boys and girls were ill treated by their teachers in the forties and fifties, it seems important to make things clear.) There was, however, one incident which left me guilt-racked for a long time – and even now it's hard to write about it. I was sitting doodling at the back of the class one day when the teacher spotted me and demanded that I bring up to her whatever it was I was doing. I knew at once that I was in deep trouble because I had been drawing the stamp on the envelope containing a letter to my best friend René. It wasn't the stamp but the contents of the letter which was the trouble. 'Dear René,' it said, 'let us go away on holiday together, but before you go, will you send me a photograph of your tummy button?' When the teacher suggested that I read the letter to the class I hung my head in shame so she took it from me and read it quietly to herself.

The year was around 1945 and I don't think that my teachers had studied much child development. Clearly they interpreted my eight-year-old fantasy as indicative of moral corruption and I was sent immediately to see the headmistress who isolated me from the rest of the school. I remember vividly how she told me to write down any other dirty thoughts that I had had. I can see to this day her propelling pencil which she had given me to write with and remember wondering if I should admit to my drawings of excretion in which pee was labelled 'lemonade' and poo 'sausages'. I don't remember what I wrote but I know that my father was sent for and I was nearly expelled as a source of moral danger to the other children. It's all so silly and so sad but it taught me early on that my body and its functions were not only dirty but something to be ashamed of.

This early learning was reinforced by my next convent school, where, as boarders, we had to put our knickers on under the bed covers in the morning lest anyone view our nether regions. The rest of our dressing was carried out face turned towards our lockers and body shrouded in a dressing gown. All this secrecy conducted under the guise of modesty inevitably left me ashamed of my body and ill prepared for sexual encounter or any kind of nakedness. I was definitely not one of the 'naughty' convent girls who leaped over the traces the moment they left school.

Some time after the letter episode my parents took me away from the convent and sent me to Cirencester grammar school where I was very much happier. A year later, however, all our lives changed radically because my father decided that we should uproot ourselves and seek our fortune in Australia, the land of his birth.

2

TEN-POUND POMS: 1949

In 1949, when I was twelve years old, my parents, my brother and I emigrated to Australia, leaving behind my sister Margaret who was pregnant with her first child. We emigrated as 'ten-pound Poms', as the Australians described those British who had their fares paid by the government if they paid the first ten pounds. The journey by sea took around six weeks and, having the run of the ship, I made friends with all manner of people. To their parents' delight, I rounded up all the smaller children and played school with them, casting myself in the role of bossy teacher and them, of course, as my obedient pupils.

Disembarking in Sydney, we made our way by car to Queensland and the Darling Downs where my parents hoped to buy a farm. This was my father's birth place and we met our Australian relatives for the first time. We stayed for a while with my Aunt Maud, who I remember as an unhappy woman who had been left with two small boys when her aristocratic English husband deserted her. The two boys farmed and for a while my father and brother helped them, but no suitable farm was found and we decided to move south. I had a great time, riding a gentle horse called Swaggy whom I loved passionately until he left me stranded one day after breaking his bridle away from the tree where I had tethered him. I always think of Swaggy when I hear Banjo Paterson's famous lines:

> 'Only a pound,' said the auctioneer,
> 'Only a pound, and I'm standing here
> Selling this animal gain or loss –

Only a pound for the drover's horse?
One of the sort that was ne'er afraid,
One of the boys of the Old Brigade;
Thoroughly honest and game I'll swear,
Only a little the worse for wear . . .'

From 'In the Droving Days' by Banjo Paterson, in
The Man from Snowy River and Other Verses (1985)

My parents searched hard for a property to buy but were disappointed and resolved to return to the UK. We said our goodbyes, therefore, and set off on the long journey south.

Once in New South Wales, however, my parents bought a five-acre poultry farm with a stock of two thousand free-range chickens and for the next ten years we played at being poultry farmers. Although we made very little money we were happy enough in our new outdoor life, though my mother always yearned for Devon, her own family and my sister Margaret who had remained in England with her husband and new baby. I was by now thirteen and was sent to school once more at the local convent, Our Lady's Convent, in Paramatta, while my brother and my parents worked on the farm.

My six years at the convent were really happy for I loved the nuns and my work flourished. By the age of fifteen I had decided against a career as a dress designer and, madly in love with the family doctor, insisted that I wanted to do medicine. My father, always an ambitious man, was delighted and supported me enthusiastically. The next two years were hard graft as I struggled with the maths and chemistry that were a requirement for entry into medical school and I had to repeat my final year because my grades were not good enough. Furiously (having burned my books and, no doubt, my school hat) I returned to school to re-sit my A levels, and it was during this year that I had my first major spiritual crisis.

For those unfamiliar with the culture of Roman Catholicism in the 1950s I should explain that it was a time when 'vocations' to the priesthood and the religious life were at their peak. The seminaries were full of enthusiastic young men, and Catholic girls, intent upon serving God in teaching, nursing or social work, entered the convents in droves. The novices, in their long black habits and white veils, were a familiar yet mysterious sight at school and led to much speculation and a certain amount of nervous tittering as we wondered who from our class would 'enter'.

It was the custom in those days for the fifth-formers (the top of the school) to make a three-day retreat and the theme that year (1955) was 'Vocations'. The school was filled with posters bearing messages such as 'We grow like those with whom we live – the nun lives with Christ' and 'Is God calling YOU to the Religious life?' At first I took no particular notice of these invitations but halfway through the retreat I began to wonder if perhaps they were addressed to me. I was appalled; much as I liked the nuns it had never crossed my mind to emulate them, after all I was going to get married and be a famous doctor and have dogs and a house and, just possibly, a couple of children. Curiously enough, I never understood this as a call to life in the missions where I could have combined medicine and religious life to great effect. Instead, I heard it as a call to abandon my dream of medicine for the cloister and I could not have been more miserable.

I did not dare to tell my parents but took counsel instead with one of the nuns and later with a priest I met in the house of a friend. No one tried to influence me in any way, but they told me to go on listening and praying that God's will should become clear to me. The novelist Antonia White, writing of her own convent school days, speaks of children contracting 'The Divine Measles', a passing affliction of 'vocationitis', before they left school to begin their lives in earnest. For me, however, this was no passing malady but a kind of itch which troubled me intermittently over the next twenty-five years until, desperate to do what was asked of me, I entered a Cistercian convent at the age of forty-one.

Now, in my late sixties, I look back to my school days and wonder what on earth was going on. Why was I so God-struck while my friends went happily on to court, marry and have children? My best friend at school went on with me to do medicine, married her anaesthetist suitor and bore him six children as well as being a top-notch occupational health physician, an ardent botanist and a connoisseur of Oriental carpets. So: why me? Was I really called by God or was it all a figment of my imagination, a religious 'complex' of some kind? One answer to my question is that I was especially ambitious spiritually. We were taught quite clearly at school that the highest possible vocation, the most generous way of serving God, was in the priesthood or the religious life. There was no question in the nuns' minds that the married state was second best, as was medicine, nursing, teaching or any other kind of good works. My father, a powerful influence in my life, was extremely ambitious for me, not, I suspect, for my happiness but that I should be successful, whatever that meant. (Perhaps he equated success and its monetary rewards with happiness.) When, many years later, he found out about my intentions to be a nun he was devastated and did everything he could to dissuade me, while I, pious little prig that I was, told him that I must obey God's holy will!

Now, in a different time with a different theology, I no longer see the priesthood and the religious life as the highest possible calling. I see religious vocation as something special but no holier than the married state or indeed the single one. Holiness, I believe, is a matter of our relationship with God and how we live out our own particular calling, whatever that may be. Medicine has been for me a deeply spiritual way of life, filling me with wonder and awe and providing a lifetime's opportunity for gospel living. Now that I no longer minister to people physically I have a deep sense of Emmanuel, God with us, as I listen to my psychotherapy clients. It is very humbling to be entrusted with another person's story, especially if he or she is deeply troubled by what has happened in the past. This work feels to me akin to priestly ministry and I feel privileged to do it.

When I hear of arrogant or abusive behaviour by Catholic priests I am filled with fury at a church which clings to the vision of an all-male and celibate clergy. I know many good and wise Catholic priests who have lived their lives as fully as possible in the service of God and his people but I find them no wiser or holier than the many married Anglican priests, men and women, who are also my friends.

When the retreat ended I threw myself back into my school work but I worried a great deal about my 'vocation' and eventually sought out a kindly priest, Father John King, who was then chaplain at the University of Technology in Sydney. Father John was a member of the Missionaries of the Sacred Heart congregation and lived in a massive ecclesiastical building in the Sydney suburb of Kensington. I remember to this day how scared I felt climbing the steps up to the monastery front door and how enormously kind he was to me. I don't recall a lot of what he said but I know he listened well, teased me gently and told me to make no decisions while my heart was in such turmoil.

At Christmas the school year ended and I did well enough in the exams to be awarded the vital grant to go to medical school. I also won first prize in an essay competition run by a local bank and entitled 'When I leave School'. In it I wrote with some passion of my vision of medicine and the judges declared themselves suitably impressed by my idealism. With hindsight, of course, medicine has been my vocation: an enormously powerful calling which has sustained me through nearly fifty years of work and study. There were few doctors in our immediate family but the ancient Cassidys of Fermanagh in Northern Ireland were hereditary physicians to the Maguires, the ruling class. I knew quite clearly from the age of fifteen that I wanted to do medicine, and have literally never looked back. The practice of it has brought me endless joy and fulfilment over the years for I have always loved the relationships with my patients and been endlessly challenged by the problems of diagnosis. When told of a medical dilemma my nose twitches in excitement like Miss Marple's and my brain slips quietly into gear. Although never really an academic, I have been endlessly fascinated by the human body and what goes wrong with it and delight in explaining how it works to anyone who will listen. Luckily for me there is a fairly constant supply of nurses eager to learn about cancer and the various kinds of emotional loss which accompany it, so I still teach regularly in the local hospice, work which keeps me on my toes intellectually and, happily, also pays for the dog food.

So where is God in this very ordinary activity: or does God have nothing to do with teaching nurses about constipation or bereavement? My understanding is that God is deeply involved in all we do and the boundary between the sacred and the profane is very blurred indeed. The gospel message is that we should love our neighbour and love has many faces. Love demands compassion and empathy but it also seeks truth, justice and reconciliation. It calls us to care for the sick, the widow and the children, not to mention the foreigner, the refugee and the asylum-seeker. It bids us be peacemakers, to beat our swords into ploughshares and work for the establishment of the Kingdom.

Just where we find God in any given activity or walk of life is part of the mystery of life, but we may rest assured that God has pitched her tent among us.

3

SANCTA SOPHIA COLLEGE: 1956

In 1956 the University College of Sancta Sophia in Sydney was run by the nuns of the Society of the Sacred Heart and housed sixty Catholic women undergraduates. I came up with several from school, in particular Ann Burn and Catherine Duncan, who were to become lifelong friends. The principal of the college was a delightful elderly nun called Mother Macrae who governed her charges with a quiet authority.

In these days of co-ed schools and teenage sex it is hard to believe how innocent most of us were. The only exposure to boys to be had at boarding school was the annual fifth-year students' ball where we were inspected individually by the nuns who firmly covered any visible cleavage with a lace handkerchief. To arrive, therefore, at college where the front door was open until ten or eleven at night and the nearest men's residence just next door felt like being dropped off in heaven. Having said this, I should make it clear that the nuns were at pains to keep us chaste. Men were not allowed in the women's rooms but had to await their friends in a small parlour known as the 'man trap'. The story in those days was that Mother McCarthy, the diminutive and elderly nun who answered the door, once showed the parlour to a prospective student's parents saying, 'And this is where the St Johns boys have intercourse with the Sancta girls.'

My first year in medical school was full and happy. There were six hundred students in that first year and we attended lectures and laboratory sessions on the main university campus. Ann and I had to work particularly hard as, unlike the boys, we had not done physics at school and had to cram five years' work into one. Like all students we worked and played to our limits; some lost their virginity and others, like myself, hung on to it. These were, of course, the pre-pill years and I doubt that abortions were legal.

At college we were encouraged, though not obliged, to attend daily Mass and I, like my friends, staggered along the corridor bleary-eyed with my black academic gown covering pyjamas or nightgown. The rest of the time, however, I was immersed in the excitement of a new life and all thoughts of being a nun were very much on the back burner. The following year, however, things were very different, for the principal, Mother Macrae, was replaced by a younger and much more assertive woman, Yvonne Swift, known to us all as Swifty.

Yvonne Swift was no mean personality. She had qualified as a lawyer before entering the convent and the story was that she had entered at midnight in full evening dress after a summer ball. Even before I had a chance to get to know her, I felt terribly challenged by her presence. Here was a woman much cleverer than I who had abandoned a high-powered career to follow Christ. She was for me the perfect role model and I was terrified.

It is hard to explain to those not brought up Roman Catholic the notion that a man or woman might not *want* to become a priest or a nun but still feel *called* to abandon career, lovers and children for the sake of Christ. The phrase 'fools for Christ' covered such people: men and women whose love for God was so huge that they had no options but to follow the Master. For me, therefore, there was no refuge in saying that I hated the idea of being a nun because this resistance could be taken as a sign of my true vocation.

Some time during that second year, Mother Swift learned of my dilemma and decided I must be helped to face what God was asking of me. She was a deeply spiritual woman and I came to love and respect her but, in hindsight, I think that she perhaps tried too hard to influence me. My memory is that she as good as told me that I had a clear vocation to the contemplative life and that I should abandon medicine and join the Society of the Sacred Heart at the end of my third year.

I was, once again, thrown into anguish and confusion and I worried endlessly about what was the right thing to do. The months, however, passed and I was deeply absorbed in my life as a medical student, dissecting cadavers and learning the intricacies of human biochemistry.

Some time during that second or third year Mother Swift arranged that the members of the college should make a three-day retreat. Separated from all distraction, I prayed and worried what I should do, torn between my desire to be generous in my following of Christ and my longing to become a doctor.

I should explain that, for whatever reason, medicine has never been just a job for me, but a passionate romance. I've always said that medicine is a whore who tolerates no rivals, and that's how it has been all my life. Small wonder that the thought of abandoning it filled me with terror.

During the course of the retreat we were offered the opportunity of some private conversation with the retreat-giver, a Father Eric D'Arcy (later to become Bishop of Tasmania). Impressed by his talks, I decided to seek his advice, only to find a queue of other students waiting patiently in line. Never a woman to stand humbly in line, I retired to the garden and hid behind a bush awaiting the priest's arrival. Sure enough, he soon strode purposefully down the path, black and white football scarf swinging round his neck and a little song on his lips. Unashamed, I leaped out from behind my bush and muttered that I needed to talk to him and that I wasn't prepared to wait in line with all those other silly women. Highly amused, he led me past the waiting students and into the 'parlour' where he was seeing people and asked me what was wrong.

Out it all poured: my longing to be a doctor and the terrible problem of 'vocationitis' that threatened to drag me screaming into a convent and leave me to drown in a sea of black-clad women. What Eric thought of this desperate young medical student I shall probably never know, but he calmed me down and repeated the famous Jesuit advice that one should never make important life-changing decisions when one's heart is in turmoil.

I walked out of the interview room a different person. Here was a priest telling me that I didn't have to be a nun: or anyway not yet. The pressure was gone and I relaxed into being myself: a slightly scatty enthusiastic young woman on the way to becoming a doctor.

Towards the end of my third year at Sancta my parents, wearying of the egg business and homesick for England, family and friends, decided to return to the UK. I was devastated. How could they abandon me, leave me behind like that? They, quite reasonably, had assumed that I was happy at Sancta, and, after all, I was being educated at the State's expense. I would have none of it and insisted on returning with them to England, so my father set about finding me a place in a British medical school. Oxford, of course, was his first choice as he himself had studied there. By great good chance the sister of an old flame of his was by then bursar at Somerville, one of the four women's colleges at Oxford. The head of the college at that time was a medical woman, the haematologist, Dame Janet Vaughan, so perhaps she was easily persuaded to take on the medical student daughter of a distinguished former Rhodes scholar. Whatever the reason, Somerville promised me a place on condition that I passed my third-year exams in Sydney. Consider, then, my dismay when I failed my anatomy exam just before we were due to sail.

There was nothing for it but to stay behind and work furiously for the re-sit of the exams in a couple of months' time. So, work I did, frantically committing to memory the names and courses of the innumerable blood vessels and nerves in the human body. Ironically, today's medical students are required to study very little anatomy and are no longer exposed to the formalin-disguised smell of death in the dissecting room. With hindsight I'm glad to have been forced to learn as much anatomy as I did, for it makes the understanding of the failing body infinitely easier.

Working through the anatomy demonstrators and technicians, I made it known to the authorities how much hung on my passing this exam and, to my utter delight, I did. Meeting the awe-inspiring professor of anatomy, 'Black-Mac', one day I thanked him profusely for letting me pass, at which he fixed me with a beady eye and said, 'You passed, Miss Cassidy, not by this much, nor this much, but by *that* much!' pressing his thumb and forefinger together until there was no space between them.

Thanking my lucky stars, I scuttled off to pack my bags, and shortly after my twenty-first birthday I left the sunburned country for the land of my birth.

4

THE OXFORD
UNDERGRADUATE:
1957

In October 1957 I presented myself at Somerville College and was sent to meet my tutor, a pint-sized Scots dynamo by the name of Jean Bannister. It didn't take me long to realise that reading medicine at Oxford was going to be very different from the way it was in Sydney. The main difference was that we were treated as adults and not as sixth-formers and were expected to derive our knowledge from original scientific papers rather than lecture notes or textbooks. I had a heavy cold that first day and was feeling lost and miserable *before* I met Miss Bannister, let alone after she'd done with me! Her final instructions were that I should go to the Parks Road to meet my other tutor, Dr Tom Parsons. When I rather pathetically asked her where the Parks were she snorted and said briskly, 'Buy a map'. The other thing, which nearly undid me, was that all college staff addressed me as 'Miss Cassidy', making the clear and completely fallacious assumption that I was grown up.

The anatomist was a gaunt middle-aged man whose first question to me was 'How are you adjusting to Oxford men, Miss Cassidy?' My answer, alas, has escaped my memory but I can still sense the disbelief at his question. Scared witless by this new world, I sought refuge in religion and was soon a regular Mass-goer, first of all at the parish church of St Aloysius next door to the college and later at the spartanly beautiful Dominican Church, Blackfriars, in St Giles.

The following week I was sitting studying in my room when there was a knock at the door; when I called 'Come in' there appeared a young man with the longest eyelashes I had ever seen. He greeted me warmly, telling me that he was the representative from the Catholic University Chaplaincy and that I would be most welcome there. Entranced by the eyelashes, I agreed to come the following Sunday, little knowing that the Chaplaincy was to become my home from home.

The chaplain that year was Monsignor Valentine Elwes, a tall and aristocratic man who looked much at home in the fifteenth-century bishop's palace which stands in St Aldates, opposite the gate to Christchurch Meadow. Father Val, as he was known, was available to see undergraduates by appointment and provided a daily Eucharist for anyone who wished to attend. His assistant was a spare and studious Belgian priest called Yves Nolet, Père Yves to the students. My initial contact with the Chaplaincy was at Mass on Sundays and I found a merry group of young men and women, many of whom seemed to have come from the well-known Benedictine schools, Downside and Ampleforth.

Most of my church-going that year was to Blackfriars, which was much nearer Somerville and I went most days to both Mass and Compline, the last monastic service of the day. Compline was sung by the friars in Latin plainchant and I found the sound of their voices magical. I have always loved plainchant and to this day it fills me with a feeling which is impossible to describe. It is as though my heart is a bell and the sound of the music sets up a vibration within me.

My second year at Oxford, however, brought me into contact with a most remarkable man, Valentine Elwes' successor as Catholic chaplain, Father Michael Hollings. Our first meeting took place in the Somerville sanatorium where I was languishing with bronchitis. One day, when I was feeling particularly lonely and miserable, there appeared a tall priest with a long nose and a kindly smile who said he was the new Catholic chaplain and how was I feeling?

'Overwhelmed' was the true answer because I couldn't believe that anyone would care enough about me to search me out like that. From that day on I was Michael's devoted disciple and we remained friends until his death in 1997. Michael Hollings became a legend in his own lifetime and, had he not been so outspoken in his views and radical in his lifestyle, might well have become Cardinal Archbishop of Westminster. Michael was of aristocratic stock and had been badly wounded during the war while serving in the Guards. It was after this that he decided to become a priest and was sent (he said) by mistake to the Beda College in

Rome, the seminary for late vocations, where he got away with four years' training rather than the usual six.

Michael was greatly influenced by Padre Pio, a famous Italian priest who was said to have the stigmata, the mystical imprint of the wounds of Christ, upon his hands. Padre Pio spent his latter years in prayer and in hearing confessions and Michael visited him a number of times at the Capuchin convent in Foggia. Michael was for me an icon figure, a human being whose transparency gives one a glimpse of the Divine.

His first term in Oxford changed the Catholic Chaplaincy for ever, for Michael's style could not have been more different from Father Val's. The first change came when he declared the Chaplaincy open house to under- graduates and provided free afternoon tea daily at four o'clock. Michael was actually quite a shy man and he would sit at his desk working in the upper room at The Old Palace while his charges talked to each other or just had their tea. The sight of him at that and subsequent desks and the sound of his voice on the telephone, 'Oxford 47870', are etched perma- nently on my memory because, for twenty or more years, he was the man who was always there for me when I was confused, miserable or in trouble. Not that he was always loving or patient: there were times when he could be sharp and critical and in his later years I was more wary of him. Having said that, I always knew that, whatever wrong I had done, whatever mess I was in, Michael would not turn me away.

In my Oxford days, of course, we were both young, I in my early twenties and Michael, I think, in his thirties. After getting to know him, I transferred my allegiance from Blackfriars to The Old Palace and came daily to the 7.40 a.m. Mass which Michael celebrated in the Nissen hut chapel which was tacked on to The Old Palace, the home of the chaplain. It was during these early morning visits to God and his local representa- tive that I learned how to pray in earnest. It happened like this: whenever I arrived a little early for Mass, Michael would be seated in his chair by the altar, quite still and apparently lost in prayer. Intrigued by the sight of him, I came each day a little earlier and sat in my chair gazing at him and the altar and trying to pray. Eventually I took to coming before 7 a.m. and waiting for him to open the chapel, after which he went to his seat and I to mine and we sat in companionable silence waiting upon God.

Later on, Michael gave a series of talks on prayer, but I don't remem- ber what he said, only the early mornings of watching and waiting. What I think I learned from Michael at quite a young age was that prayer is keeping company with God and is much more about listening than about talking. The most helpful instruction I ever received was from a

Benedictine monk who wrote, 'Pray as you can and not as you can't!' The art of listening to the Divine, to the Mystery, is of course the work of a lifetime and it takes a while to learn to relax into it. Stillness of body and mind are the main tools which prepare us for prayer without words – for listening prayer – but after a while we can learn to weave it into daily life, so that all manner of events and encounters can trigger an exchange with God. The unknown fourteenth-century author of *The Cloud of Unknowing* talks about little darts of love with which one pierces the mysterious 'cloud' where, so we believe, God dwells.

These 'little darts of love' are, for me, closely connected with my sense of wonder: that childlike delight in people and nature which causes my heart to sing. This morning I sat watching a squirrel as he leaped from branch to branch and then swung hand over fist along a wire to where his corn cob hung so temptingly. Later he ventured onto the forbidden territory of the bird-feeder, by way of a death-defying leap from the high wire to the trough. Some might find these antics a distraction but for me they are a source of endless delight and therefore gratitude. I don't actually say 'Bless you, Lord, for creating this enchanting beast, please keep it safe from marauding hawks and people'. To articulate these words in full feels unnecessary: God knows my rising and my lying down and sees me and his squirrel along with the rest of creation. All we need is a glance, a sigh, a smile to communicate, as do today's youth with their texts: 'O Gd I lv u', or just plain 'Gd'!

What gave Michael's prayer validity to me was the way he lived his life and cared for people. It wasn't just the constant availability, night and day, to us 'his' flock, but the way he loved the poor and the broken. This is straight gospel stuff and I have no time for religion without it. From the beginning of his tenure at Oxford, Michael provided tea and sandwiches to anyone who knocked at his door and at Christmas he gathered all the lonely and the odd to celebrate Christmas with him. I participated in many of these dinners and helped to welcome Michael's motley collection of ex-convicts, lonely dons and the mentally ill who gathered around the old oak table in the Chaplaincy dining room.

Michael was one of those Christians who had genuinely made a 'preferential option for the poor', as the Latin American Bishops phrased it, and, while many of us found this inspiring, it could also be quite scary (and to be truthful, rather tiresome). I became aware of this many years later when I visited Michael in his Bayswater (London) parish of St Mary of the Angels. It was my custom to spend the night at St Mary's whenever I came to London and I would arrive around nine or ten at night.

Sometimes Michael would be there and I would be warmly welcomed and feel greatly loved and cherished; at other times, however, Michael would be out and there would be two or three young men slumped in front of the television. Who these people were I never really knew except that they were people whom Michael was helping: drug addicts, unhappy seminarians, visiting African clergy and so on.

At each visit I would be invited to spend some time with him in his office, with Thomas his enormous and devoted tabby cat purring away on his desk, or beside it. Wherever he was, his office was Michael's home, the desk piled high with unanswered letters, an open box of his books among other papers filed conveniently on the floor. Slung over a chair or sofa was the black cloak which kept him warm in church, still lined with the scarlet cotton which my friends and I had hand sewn in when we borrowed it to wear to an Oxford ball. Hung over the desk was a sign declaring 'Bless this Mess', and I loved the chaos of the room, feeling safe and 'held' by its owner despite minute-by-minute interruptions of our conversation by the ever-ringing telephone.

As far as I know, Michael always slept in his office too, either on the floor or some invisible put-you-up bed. His was a simple life but one in which his radical poverty was largely hidden. To those who met him he was a cultured upper-middle-class man who enjoyed good food, wine and conversation as much as anyone, but those of us who knew him reasonably well knew that he rose at four to pray each day and made himself available until midnight or later to anyone in need.

I have written at some length about Michael because he was so enormously important to my understanding of what the spiritual life was about. It wasn't until I got to know the Jesuits many years later that I realised that Michael was what is called a contemplative in action; that is, his active life of constant giving was fuelled by a particularly rigorous life of prayer. This understanding of the Christian life has been central to my own spirituality though I have never achieved anything like Michael's enormous generosity to God and his people.

During my second pre-clinical year I continued to be a regular church-goer, attending Mass daily at the Catholic Chaplaincy and Compline at 9.00 p.m. at the Dominican church, Blackfriars. This was my first intro-duction to men religious and to the Divine Office and I was entranced by the liturgy which was so different from Sunday Mass in Australia or even at the Chaplaincy. Blackfriars is a particularly beautiful church, furnished in the simplest of styles: plain stone and clear glass. At the back of the church were chairs for the congregation while at the front was the altar with tall silver candlesticks and the massive clear-glass windows above it. The friars' choir stalls face each other across a black and white tiled stone floor.

Anyone who has never attended the monastic office of Compline has missed one of the most moving examples of Christian worship. The service is a simple one in which a hymn is followed by three psalms, always the same, and then a short reading, some prayers, the Lord's Prayer and lastly a hymn to the Virgin. The unaccompanied Gregorian chant was for me a powerful stimulus to prayer and I would usually stay quietly in my seat until it was time to lock up the church. That, I think, must have been how I met Father Peter Worrall, the next person to accompany me on my faith journey. In those days I was only too ready to bare my soul to a kindly priest so I told Father Peter about the persistent and tiresome sense of being called to a religious life which had dogged my footsteps for the past five or so years. He listened attentively and, after a while, suggested that he introduce me to the enclosed Dominican Sisters at Boar's Hill, on the outskirts of Oxford.

It was at that point that I began to panic. It was one thing to talk about religious life in general but something else to be introduced as a possible candidate. The notion of enclosed convents too made me deeply fearful and I muttered quickly that I wasn't ready. Later on, however, I agreed to visit the 'active' Dominican Sisters in Stone in Staffordshire and it was there that I met Sister Mary Mark, the headmistress of St Dominic's Convent School and sister to a well-known Dominican preacher, Father Sebastian Bullough.

Sister Mary Mark was a delightful woman: intelligent, forthright and down to earth. We talked about her own experience of entering and her horror at finding the pyjamas she had brought from home mysteriously replaced by a white flannel nightgown. Sister Mary Barbara, the red-cheeked Latin teacher, also became my good friend and I felt extremely comfortable with these women: so comfortable that, with very mixed feelings, I made a decision to enter at Stone after the completion of my first degree instead of going on to do my clinical studies.

It was with enormous trepidation that I wrote to inform my parents that I had decided to abandon my career in medicine to become a nun. Although I knew at the time that they would not welcome my decision, I had no idea that they would be as upset as they were. Each of my parents wrote to me, my father begging that I should continue in medicine where I could be 'seen to be doing good to God and man' and my mother icily commenting upon the waste it would be of my life. With hindsight, this provided the first major opportunity for me to resist my father's attempts to control my life and, delighting in the opportunity for rebellion, I wrote a polite letter back, informing them with greater than usual priggishness that I understood their distress but felt obliged to do God's holy will!

God, of course, always has the last laugh and, to my enormous surprise, I soon fell madly in love for the first time in my life. The object of my desire was Michael, a fellow medical student and a good Catholic boy: he, in fact, of the long curly eyelashes whom I had met during my first days at Somerville. Desperately confused, I sought help from my Dominican friends: the men, of course, because in those days I believed that men were wiser than women. This time my mentor was Father Sebastian, Sister Mary Mark's brother: a larger than life motorcycle-riding Dominican who would tuck his habit into his trousers and roar off to give a retreat at the other end of the country. Sebastian was wonderful and clearly understood my plight, rejoicing for me at the experience of being in love. As fate would have it, however, I had mistaken Michael's natural charm for affection and a few weeks later his best friend Tim broke it to me that Michael was engaged to be married! I was heartbroken and Tim carried me off to Michael Hollings who had clearly had experience in comforting broken-hearted undergraduates.

With hindsight, I see how immature and inexperienced I was, despite my twenty-three years. I had never really had a proper boyfriend and had certainly never had sex. I had had a couple of beaux in Sydney: David, the beautiful architect, and, later, Martin, a Catholic doctor whom I fell for three days before I was due to fly to the UK. We corresponded for a while and then he happened to visit Oxford so I was sure that our romance would blossom. He picked me up from college on a beautiful summer's evening and we wandered round Oxford's glorious inhabited ruins while I fantasised over the dinner à deux which I assumed was to follow. The night wore on and Martin made no mention of food until I declared miserably that I was completely starving. Surprised, he smiled and led me to a hot dog van and purchased me a sandwich with all the trimmings. I was not impressed, and somehow after that I didn't find him quite so attractive!

Curiously enough, after Michael of the long eyelashes had broken my heart, it never occurred to me to pursue a life with the Dominican Sisters. Perhaps I had caught the scent of ether and nothing could deflect me from embarking upon my training in clinical medicine; it was to be a full ten years before I gave any further thought to a religious call.

5

~⚬⚭~ ⚭⚬~

PLAYING DOCTORS:
1960

After obtaining their first degree many of the Oxford graduates moved to London to do their clinical studies at one of the famous medical schools such as Guys, St Thomas's or Barts. After only two years in Oxford, however, I had no desire to leave and I became part of an exceptionally small student intake of six into the Oxford medical school. There was Julian Jack, a very gifted New Zealand physiologist; Angus Campbell, a debonair Scotsman who had spent some time in the USA; John Bosco Gabriel Trouern Trend; David Evans and Ray Williams. We were split into two groups of three and I was assigned to be with Julian and Angus who became my constant companions and close friends for the next three years. The British medical clinical training at that time was based largely upon a system of apprenticeship: we were attached for up to six months at a time to a medical or surgical team, or 'firm', consisting of a 'consultant', or specialist, and around three doctors in training. Our first firm was a medical one, headed by the Regius Professor of Medicine, the eminent physician Professor Sir George Pickering. Although greatly in awe at first, I grew very fond of him and learned from him much that was to shape my future practice of medicine. Sir George was a stickler for the practice of medicine as an art and we were taught to observe and examine our patients as well as eliciting their stories (history) with infinite care. Although a scientist and a man of letters he hated medical jargon and insisted we use simple words like 'blue' instead of 'cyanosed' or 'indigestion' in lieu of the more impressive 'dyspepsia'. We were taught, too, the importance of the patient's story in making a diagnosis – an art which stood me in good stead years later when I worked in a poorly equipped clinic in Santiago and had very little opportunity to order investigations. I have always loved the art of diagnosis which I find akin to the process of detection in a murder enquiry.

My six months on Sir George's firm passed quickly and I soon stopped being afraid of him. His ward rounds, however, were always stressful as he brought with him an entourage of extremely bright doctors who worked in his research department. They clearly felt that the students were there to be baited, and vied with each other in asking us abstruse questions. I raised a laugh but scored no academic brownie points when taken unawares by the professor's question: 'Miss Cassidy! Do pregnant women get breathless?' Without thinking I answered, 'I don't know sir! I've never been pregnant!'

Our next three months were spent attached to a surgical firm and I have embarrassed memories of being sent for the first time to examine a young man's abdomen. After he had exposed his belly I touched it with a tremulous hand, enquiring as professionally as I could, 'Does that hurt?' To my utter mortification he grinned at me and said, 'No it's lovely!'

In addition to our training on the wards we attended various lectures and tutorials designed to prepare us for the day when we would be taking responsibility for the care of our own patients. Although I have few memories of these sessions, I know that I enjoyed my clinical studies vastly more than the anatomy, physiology and biochemistry which had preceded them. I was fascinated by the different diseases which affect people and I loved talking to patients, comforting them and trying to make a diagnosis.

The real excitement, however, lay in the emergency work and we joined the houseman and registrar as they examined these new and often very sick patients suffering from heart attacks, stroke, gastrointestinal haemorrhage, diabetic coma and so on. The best time 'on take' (receiving emergencies) was at night, when the flow of cases subsided at about 2 a.m. and we were brought bacon and eggs from the hospital kitchen to sustain us for further labour. Some years later I worked in emergency medicine in Leicester and would happily have made that my career were it not for the fact that I found it almost impossible to sleep during the day and as I grew older I found it increasingly difficult to function without sleep.

The Oxford medical school was an exciting place to train because, being a provincial hospital, we had a wide range of patients and diseases, unlike, so it was said, the more specialist London hospitals. The other reason was that Oxford had more than its share of academic physicians and surgeons and we were taught in small groups by some very famous men (and occasionally, women). I remember noting with some pride that not a week went by without there being a learned article by one of our teachers in either the *Lancet* or the *British Medical Journal.*

I was not as bright as Julian or Angus but made up for lack of intellectual brilliance with an excess of enthusiasm and a good bedside manner. One of the hardest things as a medical student is the learning of a number of practical skills such as venepuncture, and aspiration of fluid out of the various body cavities. Students in Plymouth's new Peninsula medical school practise these skills on state-of-the-art latex dummies – but, alas for our patients, they were our only practice materials. One of the most basic of medical procedures is the giving of various fluids including blood directly into the vein: a life-saving treatment for patients suffering from haemorrhage or dehydration. There was, therefore, no future in admitting defeat and my patients frequently ended up with a series of 'Cassidy bumps' on their forearms: bruises where I had failed to find the vein. Eventually, however, I mastered the technique and achieved minor acclaim many years later for succeeding in cannulating the big toe of a seventeen-stone woman by putting her in a hot bath for half an hour so that her only visible vein became possible to access.

In my third year at Oxford I rented a two-roomed flat at 143 Walton Street and began to enjoy a more active social life. Medical students work particularly hard, with endless laboratory sessions in addition to lectures and weekly essays. At the weekends, however, we were free to play and I spent many happy hours punting on Oxford's rivers, the Isis and the Cherwell, or toasting crumpets on my fire. On Sundays I went to the 10.30 a.m. Mass at the Chaplaincy where Michael exposed us to a variety of exciting preachers from different parts of the UK. After Mass we drank coffee and then loitered outside chatting. I held regular Sunday lunch parties, gathering together a dozen or more friends who had no better offer; I collected half a crown (twelve and a half pence) from each person invited and cycled off to buy provisions; usually spaghetti, onions and tinned mince or tuna and rice. In this way I learned to cook for largish numbers, a skill which came in handy twenty years later when I entered the convent.

For three years I worked hard at playing doctors, went to church, entertained my friends and once again managed to fall in love. This time it was my tutor who was the object of my desire and I stalked him round the hospital, loitering with intent in 'Piccadilly', a sort of crossroads and square outside the doctors' dining room where people frequently passed on their way from A to B or stopped for a gossip or to read the notice-board.

Eventually one night James (not his real name) carried me off to his cottage in a nearby village and instructed me in the ways of the world. My conscience, alas, spoiled my enjoyment for I lay guiltily awake listening to the church clock chime every quarter during the night. Luckily, the guilt didn't last and though he never took me home again, it felt wonderful to have been desired, if only for a night.

Why I never managed to throw off the guilty shackles of my convent education the way so many girls did I don't quite know. Luckily my lack of a boyfriend caused me no distress, especially as I worked all day and some nights in close proximity to all manner of delightful men. In those days, when we all worked such incredibly long hours, I suspect that female colleagues saw and enjoyed a lot more of the company of these men than did their wives who saw them more often asleep than awake. I have always been at ease with my male colleagues and greatly enjoyed the mild flirtation that the relationship allowed. I remember my glee when an orthopaedic ward round came to an abrupt halt as everyone delighted in observing my newly gold painted toenails.

Medical school was fun and I had lots of friends, both men and women, whom I remember with affection forty years on.

At the beginning of 1963, my last year at medical school, England was struck by a particularly vicious winter. It rained and it snowed and the east winds blew; pipes froze and burst and life was generally miserable for everyone, except perhaps for me who was living snugly in the overheated hospital, having secured a number of student locums. When a house officer (a recently qualified doctor) is ill or takes a holiday, the posts were sometimes filled by senior medical students who, though they received no pay, were given free board and lodging and an unbeatable opportunity to learn. The other perks of these jobs was an instant increase in status so that one took one's coffee with the consultant and his team while the students kicked their heels in the corridor. I somehow managed to do a string of locums over the six weeks of the freeze and felt extremely one up on Angus and Julian.

In July 1963 I took my finals and, to my enormous delight passed; now I was really a doctor, though I would not be licensed to practise outside the hospital for another year. That night we had the medical school ball and, to my great delight, the divine James carried me aloft across the dance floor in celebration of my triumph. The day after, I woke late in my flat and lunched off some strawberries and leftover mackerel. An hour later, I developed a crashing headache and glancing in the mirror saw to my horror that my face was bright red. Convinced I must be about to have a cerebral haemorrhage, I sought out James who happened to be on emergency duty in the hospital for the weekend. He took one look at me and, laughing the while, admitted me to one of the Professor's beds and filled me with adrenaline and antihistamines. By the evening I was well enough to go home, though I must admit to weeping at the thought that I might be allergic to strawberries! It wasn't till the following summer that I dared to sample them again at an enormous medical dinner, reckoning that if I did have a reaction help would be readily at hand.

Once the festivities surrounding graduation were over, we applied for the house jobs which would become vacant on 1 August. Luckily for me Julian chose to go for a job on the professional haematological unit (where he would have alternate nights off to go home to his wife), leaving Angus and me to fight for Professor Pickering's job. We approached him together saying, 'Sir – we have a problem: we both want to do your job.' Grinning from ear to ear, the great man pointed a finger at us and said, 'I'll have you – no you!' To my utter delight he meant me and I whooped with delight – little knowing what a bitter-sweet experience it would be.

Sometime later we had formal interviews, and I went in my charcoal grey suit with nothing underneath and a rose pinned to the lapel. Professor Leslie Witts who headed the interview panel delighted me by exclaiming, 'Dr Cassidy! You look like an artist's model!' Sure enough, it was announced that I had Sir George's job, confirming James's advice to me, 'Never go for a job which hasn't been rigged in your favour!' Times, of course, have changed and interviews have to be seen to be squeaky clean, unbiased. You can't ask a woman if she's married these days, let alone who'll look after her children when they have a day off school. But this was 1963 and I, a woman in a man's world, had got the top professional job at the Radcliffe Infirmary in Oxford and I was on cloud nine!

There followed a brief holiday and then on 1 August I arrived breathless at 8 a.m. at the main door of the Infirmary. Flinging my bike against the wall, I ran through the corridors and up the stairs to Collier ward where I was to begin my new career. It was three months before I had a day off and, when I went to retrieve it, my bicycle had gone.

6

PLAYING DOCTORS
FOR REAL:
1963

I t is a standing joke in medicine for the older doctors to say to the new
recruits, 'You young people have never had it so good! Now in *my*
day . . .' I make no apology then for saying that, in my day, it was
expected that junior doctors, or 'housemen' as we were called,
would be on call for their patients twenty-four hours a day, seven days a
week. We literally had no official time off and, if we needed to leave the
hospital even for ten minutes, we had to persuade a friend to cover for us.
This was no real problem if things were quiet, but if one had a patient
likely to need urgent attention then there was simply no question of
going out. Mostly, we got enough sleep to survive, but sometimes we felt
as though we would die of fatigue. I did a brief spell on the head injury
unit and learned to nap standing up leaning against a wall. Fatigue was
the one thing which could reduce me to tears and I remember sitting in
a darkened X-ray room with the tears rolling down my cheeks as I waited
at some ungodly hour for a patient with a minor head injury to be X-
rayed.

Lack of sleep, of course, took its toll on performance. I have vivid
memories of an elderly woman with a gastrointestinal haemorrhage
whom we saved by operating on her in the middle of the night. The
following night I was rung at 2 a.m. because she had developed cardiac
asthma, a terrifying episode of acute heart failure which is often fatal.

Kneeling up on the bed I injected diuretics into her femoral vein and once more saved the day. The following night she bled again and I was called to her. I know I did my best but my heart was not in it and she died. Probably, she would have died anyway, but perhaps, if I had been fresh and rested . . .?

My first six months as a doctor were particularly hard. There were no students attached and I bore the brunt of the frustrated clinical energies of the research doctors. I remember clearly Bill Cranston, the First Assistant to the Professor and later Professor of Medicine at St Thomas's, who always seemed to think up abstruse investigations which I should have done but hadn't. To my great sadness and fury, 'James' who had been the 'registrar' – the senior doctor in day-to-day charge of the ward patients – had completed his stint and was replaced by Patrick 'Spud' Murphy, cruelly known as 'the potato'. Patrick was a clever man and a good doctor but we did not really click and he was, quite reasonably, irritated by my lack of method and organisation, a gift which I still possess. When I left, however, he presented me with a copy of *The Eating in Bed Cook Book* in which he had inscribed the message, 'Perhaps one day you'll cook me a meal!'

Apart from the sleep deprivation, I greatly enjoyed the work and became very close to the patients, especially the young ones. As an older woman I sometimes reflect upon how I became acquainted with grief and death at such an early age, but I have no memory of finding it difficult. Having said that, there are some patients whom I remember by name and how saddened I was when we lost them.

One such patient was Thomas Harrison, a man in his forties with young children who had had an abdomino-perineal resection of the rectum[1] for cancer. The wound had been left open to granulate (heal) and on the tenth post-operative day or thereabouts he had a catastrophic haemorrhage from the wound. There being no vessel to ligate, all we could do was replace the blood by transfusion and hope that the bleeding would stop of its own accord. It didn't however, and after we had given him twenty pints of rare O negative blood the transfusion laboratory said that they could not in conscience give us any more blood as they had to hold a certain amount in reserve for emergencies such as obstetric haemorrhage. After consultation with Mr Webster, the surgeon, we made the sad but inevitable decision to withdraw treatment and I was sent with David the registrar to inform his wife of our decision. We spoke to Mrs Harrison in the doctor's office, David explaining that there was nothing more we could do. There was a pause as she wept, and then, composing herself, she said, 'Would you pray with me doctor', and fell to her knees on the floor. David took one look at me, said, 'Dr Cassidy will pray with you, Mrs Harrison', and beat a hasty retreat. I was embarrassed but joined her on the floor and assented as she prayed out loud for her husband to be saved.

According to all the laws of medicine and nature, Tom Harrison should have bled to death there and then – but he didn't. After a while, the bleeding stopped and he lay there, pale and wan but very much alive. His wife was convinced it was a miracle and I was inclined to agree with her while David, even more embarrassed, muttered sceptically. Over the next few weeks, Thomas had three further major bleeds, each potentially fatal, each, however, stopping spontaneously. With hindsight we decided that he was bleeding from a major pelvic vein which stopped bleeding when loss of blood volume lowered his blood pressure to a level where the blood ceased to flow, allowing the clotting mechanism to proceed. Although we found a scientific answer to what happened, perhaps it was a miracle that we were forced to stop transfusing him because by keeping his blood pressure up we were permitting the bleeding to continue.

This drama brought me very close to Tom, especially during my management of each of the subsequent haemorrhages, as I sat beside him, running the drip ever so slowly and praying that the bleeding would stop before his blood pressure became dangerously low. Eventually, he went home and although I think the cancer returned, he had precious time with his family. Saving lives, and accompanying people as they face death, is the great privilege of the physician and I always felt the draught as the door to heaven swung closed after a death.

Not all our cases of course had such happy endings. I remember a patient of Julian's, a delightful architect who had a rare condition called the Zollinger Ellison Syndrome in which there is excess excretion of digestive acid. We had diagnosed his condition and he had survived major surgery only to perforate his gut and die just when we were congratulating ourselves that we had saved him.

About halfway through my six months' appointment as house physician to the Regius Professor I became furiously angry at the hours I was expected to work. I had had no night or weekend off for three months and I felt exploited and unappreciated. In conversation with Patrick, I let fly and then burst into tears of rage and exhaustion. This was not the way the professor's junior doctor was expected to behave, however, and Bill Cranston appeared and told me I was to have two (or was it three?) days off. There was no sympathy, no apology and I realised

I was being sent home in disgrace because I was clearly not up to the job. Furious and deeply humiliated, I departed and, having slept for three days, returned with a grim determination never to show my feelings again.

At the end of my sojourn with the Professor I took up the post of house surgeon to a wonderful teddy bear of a man called Arthur Elliot Smith. It was the most coveted surgical house job and I shared it with my good friend Julian Jack who was doing the minimum number of house jobs required for registration before disappearing for ever into the Oxford physiology labs on a fast track to a chair in neurophysiology. I enjoyed working for ES, as he was affectionately known, and during the six months learned to take out an appendix and perform a circumcision. Some of the latter turned out a bit lopsided and I have often wondered a little nervously if they ended up straight in the long run. Mr Elliot Smith was the surgeon who operated on newborn babies and it was a delight to see such gentle skill in a big man.

My friend Angus worked for the Professor of Surgery, Mr Alison, who was in charge of the Cardiac Surgery Unit. In 1963, heart surgery was relatively new and quite a number of patients died. As students we had been particularly upset about the children with severe congenital heart deformities who seemed to us to come in well and with such high hopes only to die on the table or in the early post-operative period. The fact was that they would die anyway, and surgery gave them a chance of life. I remember Angus telling us that a man in his thirties had come in for a coronary artery bypass and, after Angus had explained to him exactly what his chances were, he left the hospital smartly without talking to the professor.

Robert Alison was clearly an eminent surgeon and he too had an entourage of doctor assistants doing their master's degree in surgery. My clearest memories of the professional ward round was of the women, each clad in a special nightgown (designed by the professor), which could be easily pulled down to the waist to expose the chest. Imagine around ten surgeons, the ward sister, the physiotherapist and a handful of students all gathered round a bed while the professor examined the woman's naked chest and called upon his team to listen to some interesting heart sounds. It was an appalling and dehumanising performance and I vowed I would never subject anyone to such terrible indignity.

One of the things which has changed for the better in British medical practice is the doctor–patient relationship. When I first worked in the hospice I learned from the women with gynaecological malignancy how deeply humiliated they had sometimes been by their doctors. In the 1980s I assisted in the Gynaecology-Oncology Combined Clinic and was appalled at the subtle and unthinking ways in which the patients were dehumanised. Each woman would be placed by the nurse in the examination room, lying on the couch without her underpants and with her skirt pulled up to her waist. She would then be left, covered of course with a sheet, until the doctors came to see her. The two consultants, 'power-dressed' in their immaculate and expensive suits, would enter and with a cool politeness enquire about the woman's symptoms, after which they would, gingerly (or so it seemed to me), lift the sheet exposing the woman's nakedness from ribs to thighs. After examining the woman's abdomen came the inevitable internal examination, and the humiliation was complete.

I've no doubt that all the hospital staff involved meant well but they were totally lacking in empathy: appreciation of what it felt like to be thus treated. I remember so well a woman who had that most humiliating of cancers, carcinoma of the vulva, the external genitalia. She had had surgery which had been successful for a while, but now it was obvious to all that the disease had recurred. After the examination the woman began to cry and instead of making any effort to comfort her, the gynaecologist smiled and, placing his finger on the tip of her nose said playfully, 'Now, now Iris, we don't want any of that, do we!'

Observing behaviour of this kind fuelled the fire of my rage that patients should be treated in this way and, many years later when I was called upon to lecture on emotional distress in malignant disease, I spoke out strongly on the need to treat patients differently. Now, twenty years on, things are very different. Nurses, for so long subservient to the doctors, have found their voice and have been active in the struggle for patients' rights. The patients, too, are much more outspoken and have demanded, both singly and in groups, that they be given the respect they deserve. So many good things have happened in medicine over the past twenty to thirty years, but, for now, the year is 1964 and I am a very junior doctor in a man's world.

As we moved towards the end of our pre-registration year we discussed which specialty we would choose to follow. Julian, as I have said, intended to return to neurophysiology while Angus wanted to be a psychiatrist. In the close and intellectually snobbish circles in which we moved, medicine (as opposed to surgery) was top dog, while the specialties of oncology, ENT or public health were not even to be considered by the elite as we then saw ourselves. The time had come to leave the safety of our teaching hospital where we were known and protected and strike out in the wide world.

It was at this stage that I began to understand that I could no longer count on the reflected glory of my two brilliant colleagues and would have to stand on my own two feet. Angus received a cracking reference from the Prof and was promised a job in the department that Sir George had developed at St Mary's Hospital, Paddington. My reference was very different and went something like this: 'Sheila Cassidy was my clerk[2] and my house physician. She is a very nice girl and can present a case history in a masterly fashion.' Clearly, I was not destined for one of the great teaching hospitals! Sir George, however, got me a job with one of his friends, who, curiously enough, was also a friend of my family.

Dr Clive Sowry was a consultant physician at the Edgware General Hospital in London and pronounced himself delighted to give me a job. I spent seven months as a senior house officer with Clive and successfully broadened my grasp of clinical medicine. Clive was a specialist in the care of people with diabetes as well, being a very experienced general physician. He was also an extremely kind man as well as being a good teacher and I greatly enjoyed working for him. He in his turn delighted in my enthusiasm and willingness to fetch and carry notes, X-rays or blood results and christened me 'the Little Red Hen', from the children's story of 'The Cock, the Mouse and the Little Red Hen', because, like her, I was always rushing about doing things.

Edgware served an area with a considerable Jewish population and it took me a while to get used to a different culture. Heart disease seemed to be rampant among them and I became quite slick at treating middle-aged men with pulmonary oedema, the terrible breathlessness which occurs when the heart loses strength and the lungs fill with fluid. Initially I disliked these patients because they nearly always wanted a second opinion and I felt outraged on my boss's behalf. Clive, however, had no problem with this and told me to stop fussing. After that I grew to understand them and to my enormous delight had a tree planted in Israel in my name by a grateful patient.

During these early years as a resident doctor I was so absorbed in my new world and virtually a prisoner in the hospital that I forgot about nuns and got used to missing church. Instead, I took my fun wherever I could find it and for the year of my residency cooked supper on a Saturday night in the kitchenette off the residents' sitting room. This was the old operating theatre and was a wonderful room in which to entertain. During the week we would sometimes meet in each other's rooms in our dressing gowns to drink whisky or liqueurs at bedtime. Even with all the opportunity in the world most of us lived as brother and sister, though I must admit being rather jealous of one young woman doctor who seemed to have no morals and a great deal of fun!

After my time in Edgware I returned to Oxford to do a locum in the Accident Service and, to my enormous surprise, fell madly in love with the drama of it as well as the hands-on repair of wounds. For three months I revelled in the excitement and comradeship of a busy emergency department. When the locum came to an end, I went to the boss, a tall gentle Canadian called Big Jim Scott, and asked him if I might apply for the full six-month job. He smiled at me and said something like, 'I'm so sorry, my dear, but it's not really a job for a woman.' Sadly, therefore, I left Oxford to spend a few weeks' holiday in Devon.

I had been home for no more than a couple of days before I received a frantic phone call from the hospital personnel manager: 'Come back, come back,' he said. 'The Canadian doctor who has come to do the job says he's got six kids and a new baby and there's no way he's going to do night work!' To my utter delight I returned to Oxford where I signed a contract to work for six months as senior house officer (SHO) in the Accident Service – only the second woman doctor to do the job in living memory. Those were the days: when men were men and women were only employed if there was no man available!

NOTES
1. This radical operation involves removal of rectum and anus *en-bloc*.
2. A 'clerk' is a medical student serving his or her apprenticeship.

7

—◦◦◦◦—

MENDING BROKEN PEOPLE:
1965

The nine months I spent in the Oxford Accident Service were some of the happiest of my medical career. I loved the fast-moving nature of the work and the diagnostic challenges involved in caring for accident victims who could be stable at one moment and at death's door the next. I loved too the repair work to hands and faces cut by glass, knives or some other sharp object and became reasonably skilled in suturing and wound care in general. Two years after my stint in Oxford I did a further couple of years in the Emergency Department at the Leicester Royal Infirmary, so the patients I saw there have merged in my mind with those whom I treated in Oxford.

Each day was a new learning experience which increased my confidence as a doctor and as a person. It was a deep joy to me to use my hands as well as my head and, had my life turned out differently, I would certainly have been a surgeon. The treatment of minor fractures was part of my job and I found the realignment of displaced bones particularly satisfying.

Most of the work in A & E is, medically speaking, relatively minor – though never trivial, of course, to the injured person. Luckily, I enjoyed the minor injuries work too and took much pleasure in reassuring patients that their wounds would heal and that function would return. In Leicester I ran a daily clinic, treating and following up injuries and infections to hands and fingers. I remember well the distress of the miners who, from time to time, sustained crush injuries to the hand and would come to casualty not only in great pain but afraid that their injury would cost them their jobs. These injuries could be hard to treat because of fractures, coal dust in the wound and badly damaged tissues.

It was around this time that I thought about becoming a hand surgeon, but before I could even think about it I had to do the FRCS, the surgical fellowship exam which seemed at the time beyond my grasp. During my Oxford casualty days, I wanted nothing more than to continue working with accident victims. It is human nature to remember one's triumphs while forgetting work that was barely good enough. It is in this spirit that I recount my greatest casualty triumph which was reducing a dislocated hip. The hip joint, as you can imagine, is held together by a group of extremely powerful muscles, so the force required to displace it is considerable and reduction is usually considered a task for a beefy orthopaedic surgeon. One night in Leicester we called the anaesthetist at 4 a.m. in the morning to anaesthetise a six-foot-six man whose hip had been violently wrenched from its socket in an accident. All was well until we realised that the orthopaedic registrar was nowhere to be found. The anaesthetist, who was determined to return to his bed as soon as possible, became very irritated and said to me, 'You'll just have to do it yourself!' Nervously, I followed his instructions and standing up on the trolley took hold of the man's thigh and pulled upwards for all I was worth. To my delight there followed a dramatic clunk announcing that the head of the femur was safely back in its socket. As you can imagine, I was insufferably proud for days!

As my six months in the Oxford A & E drew to its close I knew for certain that I wanted to do surgery but feared that I might not have the physical strength required for orthopaedics and A & E. (This was before the triumph of my hip reduction!) I began, therefore, to consider whether plastic surgery might be a good alternative, and applied for the SHO post in the Oxford Plastic surgery Department at the Churchill Hospital at Headington. Plastic surgery, of course, is nothing to do with plastic: it involves the moving of skin to cover defects which may be at any place on the body. In some ways it is akin to dressmaking (at which I was adept) but in other ways it is very different because the covering of the body is not cloth but living tissue totally dependent upon its blood supply. The treatment of burns falls within the remit of the plastic surgeon who shaves incredibly fine layers of skin from undamaged areas to apply to those regions in which a full-thickness burn has destroyed the skin. Such 'split skin' grafts are life-saving, although the ultimate cosmetic result usually leaves much to be desired.

The really exciting part of plastic surgery is the long drawn-out process of moving, in stages, a full-thickness layer of skin from one end of the body to the other. Eric Peet, whose job I had applied for, was internationally famous for creating ears out of rib cartilage and the skin of the neck in children who were born with a congenital absence of the ears. Reconstruction was done in stages. First of all, a tube of skin was formed on the neck, then when this had healed one end was cut and sewn in place on the scalp where the ear was to be built. When the skin was securely attached with a good blood supply, the other end was detached and also sewn to the scalp, providing the skin from which the ear would be fashioned. These techniques were also valuable in facial reconstruction after injury or cancer surgery and I was amazed to learn that the reconstruction of the nose using the skin of the forehead was first done by the ancient Egyptians. Cosmetic work, which is how most people think of plastic surgery, was done mostly in the private hospitals, so it wasn't until I worked in Chile that I saw my first facelift. This is not the place to discuss the ethics of cosmetic surgery but there is no doubt that it brings much satisfaction to both surgeon and patient.

With my six months in the Radcliffe A & E Department coming to an end, I set out to plan my surgical career. The next stage was to be six months' plastic surgery, followed if possible by a year of general surgery at SHO level. During this time I had to study for the Primary Fellowship: the first part of the academic surgical qualification. I found the prospect seriously daunting as the examiners required (quite reasonably) an extremely detailed knowledge of anatomy, something which I had always found difficult.

My first introduction to this basic medical science had been in my second year at the University of Sydney. I don't think any medical student forgets the mixture of awe, disgust and excitement which overcomes them on the occasion of their introduction to the dissecting rooms. Only in some hideous major disaster would one contemplate a room with twenty or fifty dead bodies lying in rows: but this is the daily experience of the second- and third-year medical student. I hated dissection: the cadaver smelt and was greasy to the touch and seemed to bear little relationship to the lovely artists' drawings in my atlas in which arteries were bright red, veins deep blue and nerves yellow. In the body all these vessels looked the same and I despaired of distinguishing one from the other.

The dissecting-room experience is also the students' first encounter with the black humour which is an emotional safety valve in so much of medicine. The story I remember best is of the medical student who saw an elderly gardener working in the garden way below the dissecting room. 'Would you like a hand, dad?' the student called down. 'That would be great,' said the old man. So the student threw him down one! Such humour, while upsetting to the outsider, is one of the things which makes possible the daily encounter with tragedy and death.

The more I think about it, particularly these days when I spend a good deal of time studying anatomy and physiology in preparation for my lectures, I believe that medicine is an immensely spiritual discipline. Knowledge of how the body and the brain function fills me with awe and fascination and leaves me ever more convinced of a creator God. We live in a time of increasing enlightenment in which ever more powerful microscopes, scans and chemical techniques reveal to us in more and more depth how wonderfully we are formed, and it is no surprise to me that there are as many scientists who find their faith in God strengthened by their knowledge as there are atheists who insist that science proves there is no creator.

When my time in A & E was up I prepared to move myself and my belongings up to the Churchill Hospital in Headington where the Oxford Plastic Surgery Unit was located. To my delight and amazement, Tom Patterson, one of the consultants, suggested I should take a week's holiday before starting the new job, so I took myself off to Devon with alacrity.

The Churchill Hospital in 1966 was an extension of the Radcliffe Infirmary and housed the departments of plastic surgery, some general surgery, radiotherapy and obstetrics. The hospital was built during the war and had been handed over by the Americans to the British when they returned home. The building was strictly utilitarian: single storey with wards running off a half-open corridor arranged in the form of a square. I had visited the hospital as a medical student so was familiar with its Spartan lines but my heart sank when I was shown my room in one of two Nissen huts made from corrugated asbestos or similar material. Accommodation for resident doctors at that time was famous for being 'basic' throughout the UK, but these rooms defied belief, containing an ancient bed, a desk, some shelves and an upright chair. I was outraged at the meanness of the authorities and spent the weekend converting my bed into a divan by sawing off the head and tail boards. The following Monday I received a summons to the administrator's office where a Mr Stark accused me of damaging hospital property. As I explained my actions he enquired why on earth I hadn't requested a divan if that's what I wanted, to which I replied truthfully, 'It never occurred to me that you'd give me such a horrible bed if you had anything better!' Temporarily lost for words, he bid me goodbye, but, as things turned out, this was not to be our last encounter.

The bosses in the plastic surgery department were delightful and as different from each other as the proverbial chalk from cheese. Eric Peet was a big man, red faced and somewhat irascible. He was nearing retirement and was greatly respected for his skill as a surgeon, particularly in the repair of congenital defects in children. Tom Patterson was a younger man and very different from his senior colleague. He was always sweet tempered and a joy to work with, his humour lightening the long drawn-out operations. Tom was interested in research but did little or no private work, whereas Eric had a thriving practice at the Acland Nursing Home where the surgeons saw their private clients. My memory of Eric is that he bemoaned the meanness of his NHS salary while Tom sang as he worked and would often exclaim, 'I can't believe they actually pay me to do this.'

The third member of the team was senior registrar, John Batstone, a kind man and a meticulous surgeon who, when I went to Chile a few years later, gave me a set of plastic surgery instruments to use there. John took over the department when Mr Peet retired and Tom abandoned clinical work to become a medical historian.

A fourth member of the department in whom I had little interest at first was a shy Chilean woman in her thirties called Consuelo Silva. Consuelo was in Oxford on a British Council scholarship and it was she who had worked as locum during my recent week's holiday. Later, however, we became close friends and it was she who inspired me to seek my fortune in Chile at the end of 1971.

My memory of work as SHO in plastic surgery was that it was fairly leisurely after life in A & E. Virtually all our work was elective, that is, people were given a date to come into hospital and were operated on a few days later. Much of Eric's work was with small children: babies with cleft lip and palate; little boys with no ears and a curious condition called hypospadias in which the urinary opening in small boys did not reach to the tip of the penis but ended half way down the shaft or even at the base. The theory was that this deformity should be corrected before the boy went to primary school lest he be teased mercilessly by his companions for having to sit rather than stand to pee. The surgery was extremely fiddly, involving the creation of a tube of skin from the underside of the shaft of the penis, and it was seriously tedious to assist at, involving the holding of fine skin hooks for what seemed like hours on end. A much easier operation was the re-alignment of so-called 'bat' ears which stuck out almost at right angles from the child's head. This was the bread and butter of the paediatric work, but the adults were very different. A good deal of the work was the surgical removal of facial or oral malignancies and was done in conjunction with the facio-maxillary surgeons and the radiotherapists. My memory of these cases is that the cancer frequently recurred and the pain involved was severe, it being before the days of skilled pain control in cancer.

Whenever I had any spare time, I studied anatomy in preparation for the surgical fellowship exam, installing myself in a tiny disused laboratory which I decorated with pots and pots of hydrangeas. In the evenings the resident staff met in the doctors' mess where they played snooker and drank, talked or watched TV. It was during these evenings and particularly the long dull weekends on duty that I got to know Consuelo. We would sit in my room and gossip, finding that we had much in common, especially a love of animals, books and music. Consuelo, it turned out, was far better read than I was; she was a devotee of Evelyn Waugh, P. G. Wodehouse and Agatha Christie. She told me of her life in Chile, of her sisters Carmen and Marie Elena, and how her mother had had TB as a girl and spent a long time in a Swiss sanatorium where she had been greatly influenced by a young Communist poet. When Consuelo's mother returned to Chile she was told not to marry and certainly not to have children, but she ignored all advice and died young of TB, leaving her husband to raise their three little daughters.

Jorge Silva was devastated by his wife's death and worried that the children would follow her. Instead of sending them to school, he hired a governess and the girls became fluent in English and well versed in English literature. Consuelo grew up to be a shy girl but through her friends she developed a passion to bring justice to the poorer people of her country. She studied medicine and specialised in plastic surgery in addition to her work at the poorest of the city's four emergency hospitals, the Posta Tres, or 'Third Post'. More of this work later.

As she was not on the paid medical staff of the hospital, Consuelo was not resident and lodged with a woman in Headington where she was extremely lonely. By that time I had made friends with the other doctors in our hut, one of whom was Philomena Shaw, a psychotherapist. Phil and Consuelo and I debated what we could do until, quite by chance, we passed the last room in the hut, a storeroom, usually locked but now standing open. I grabbed Phil by the arm and pulled her in and closed the door; we surveyed the room and its contents: there was a good window, a disassembled bed, a mattress and a number of suitcases. We piled the cases up in one corner and reassembled the bed. Consuelo had a new home! She moved in there very happily, decorating the room with a rug and a small Chilean flag and we all rejoiced in our ingenuity. All was well for a few weeks but somehow we upset the cleaner who reported Consuelo to Mr Stark. The following day, Consuelo received a formal letter informing her that the box room was not suitable accommodation and she must vacate it forthwith. We were desolate, but then inspiration struck. Phil was desperately missing her husband Pete, so we calculated that if Consuelo did her night calls, Phil could take Consuelo's ancient car 'Harry' home each night and Consuelo could sleep in her vacant bed! We put this to Phil and she was delighted, driving home at around nine o'clock each night. If my memory serves me right, this regime continued until I moved on to do the general surgical SHO job and Consuelo took over as SHO in plastic surgery and was allocated a room of her own.

The surgical SHO job lasted twelve months and involved working for three surgeons: Charles Webster, a Scots colonic surgeon, Joe Smith, a urologist, and Malcolm Gough, a general surgeon. The three men were very different: Charles, I think, was in his fifties, a meticulous and caring surgeon who suffered agonies of worry after operating on high-risk patients with inflammatory bowel disease such as ulcerative colitis or Crohn's disease. He liked me to phone him every night at six o'clock precisely to report on how his patients were, so that he could switch off and relax with a good malt. Joe Smith was a younger man, endlessly sweet tempered and relaxed and a joy to work with. Mr Gough, however, took his work and himself much more seriously than the others and I had to mind my Ps and Qs. I enjoyed working for each man and learned a lot more about people and their surgical problems. Sometime in this eighteen months at the Churchill I sat the Primary FRCS, the Fellowship of the Royal College of Surgeons, but failed initially, going on to pass it the following year.

Meanwhile, in our spare time, Consuelo and I were busy trying to make our bleak hospital rooms more homely. I was a shameless skip-raider and rescued a very comfortable armchair which I covered in a bright red blanket to cheer us up. As the months passed we wearied of hospital food and one Saturday afternoon purchased a small fridge and a very small electric cooker, which, against all regulations, we installed in my room. From that time on it was 'haute cuisine' each day as we cooked steak and lamb chops doused in cognac and cream.

We were not the only homemakers in the hut. Danny, the Australian obstetric registrar, lived with his wife Elise and their baby, and Roger, another SHO, lived with his Chinese girlfriend. We did not enquire whether this cohabitation was against the rules: we knew it was, and took good care not to upset the cleaner who was our link with management. Our hours were so long and our accommodation so dreary that we felt we were in a strong position to mutiny. In fact, we came very near to making a takeover bid for a nearby new day-case unit which was being furnished with loving care and a good deal of money. Our plan was to move in the night before the public opening, but we decided against it on the grounds that the rooms, though beautifully furnished, were too pokey.

Eventually Consuelo's six months as plastic surgery SHO came to an end and she took a post in the local psychiatric hospital. This meant, of course that she was again homeless, so I obtained a mattress off the skip and arranged my room for two. The cleaners were so used to us that I don't think they even knew that she was supposed to have moved out. Our lives took a different turn, however, when Consuelo arrived home from work one day with a small green parrot whom she named Alexander. She had seen him in the pet shop in Headington and had liberated him for a better life. I was entranced but worried that maybe we were pushing our luck. Consuelo, however, who was an adept liar, convinced herself that he had been given her by a psychiatric patient and to have refused him would have had dire consequences. This began a long and complicated relationship with creatures great and small as Consuelo and I shamelessly disobeyed hospital regulations and turned our room into a zoo.

8

THE MENAGERIE EXPANDS

One day it was my turn to buy seed for Alex and I took myself off to the pet shop where I encountered and fell in love with our next room-mate, a chipmunk whom I named Henrietta. Henrietta made an entrancing companion. She was very busy and skittered about all over the room hiding caches of sunflower seeds in preparation for the winter. Luckily she always returned to her cage to sleep and to use the bathroom, although one night she decided on a sleepover and when we came to bed there was no sign of her in her cage. We searched anxiously until I noticed a small hole in my bedspread and found her happily ensconced in the mattress, having bored her way through all the bed clothes! Henrietta was also a keen gardener and I would know it was morning when she leaped onto my bed from the floor and up onto the window box where she would proceed to dig furiously, usually showering me with earth so that I was forced under the bed-clothes or out of bed.

Once we'd broken the pet-owning rule twice there seemed no reason to stop and we decided that Henrietta needed a mate. The only problem was, of course, that we didn't really know for certain whether she was male or female. Consuelo refused to be daunted and announced that she would examine Henrietta under anaesthetic. Those were the days when ether was used on the wards as a solvent, so Consuelo had no problem obtaining her anaesthetic. We had no machine, of course, and there was no way that Henrietta would be a willing participant. The goldfish bowl, however, provided an excellent solution and Henrietta was placed under it with a swab soaked in ether. At first it seemed to have no effect but then she became unsteady on her paws and keeled over. I was by this time in a state of terror that we would end up killing her and insisted that we should stop. In her soporific state we upended her; but found ourselves none the wiser! I quickly drew a diagram of her undercarriage, finishing just seconds before she leaped indignantly to her feet and shot off muttering chipmunk obscenities.

The next time I was able to escape the hospital I took myself off to the university zoology department and asked the first person I met if he could tell Henrietta's gender from my diagram. He looked puzzled and suggested we go down to the rodent quarters and compare my diagram with some of its inhabitants. The conclusion we came to was that Henrietta was indeed female, so Consuelo and I set out for the pet shop to find her a mate. The pet shop, however, had *three* baby chipmunks and, overcome by maternal lust, I bought all three. All was not well on my return, however, because Henrietta clearly did not share my feelings towards the babies and set upon them with vigour. We rescued them urgently and restored them to their cage: so now we had one very wild and possessive adult chipmunk and three frightened babies who were to become delightfully tame.

So famous did Consuelo and I become among our medical colleagues that David, who was by then plastic surgery SHO, suggested to a friend of his that we would be good people with whom to leave his two very special, rare, extra large gerbils. So that's how it was that we became the keepers of one small green parrot, four chipmunks and two very rare, very special, large, brown gerbils. The gerbils we found to be unlovely creatures but we welcomed them none the less. All went well for twenty-four hours until Gerbil A caught his tail in the door as it shut, sustaining a very impressive degloving[1] injury of the end two-thirds of his tail so that all the vertebrae were exposed. We had a medical consultation as to the best plan of action and decided that amputation was the only viable option. We went off in search of ether and surgical instruments, returning fifteen minutes later to find that Gerbil B had operated successfully on his brother who now had a neat little stump, enabling instant recognition. Foiled in our attempt at surgery we christened them instead, naming them Stumpy and Scrumpy.

As I mentioned earlier, the gerbils were not particularly good company, largely because they were nocturnal animals and spent the day asleep, unlike the chipmunks who played happily during the day and retired to bed as soon as darkness fell. Sometime after we acquired the gerbils we were due for some holiday and decamped with our entire ménage to Devon. (This was an easy journey compared with later years when we had acquired three chows as well so that the birds had to travel on the roof rack in specially windproof cages.)

This was a momentous holiday in that we lost one of the vermin and gained a parrot. Penny was a large and extremely vocal bird: a red and blue macaw whom we found for sale in the pet shop in Kingsbridge. She was the most exotic of our beasts, and lived with us until I went to Chile in 1971. Poor Scrumpy, however, came to a sticky end and was found with his little jaws clamped tightly round the electric cable at the back of the fridge.

We returned to Oxford a week later with Penny, Alexander, Henrietta and the three babies and one rather lonely large brown gerbil. Worried that Penny or the chipmunks would escape, we covered the windows with wire netting and settled down to enjoy life in our miniature zoo. The baby chipmunks were very tame and I would visit the wards with one tucked in the pocket of my white coat. As time went by, however, we worried that the powers that be would, using the cleaner's key, visit the room in our absence and take exception to our room-mates. Consuelo decided, therefore, that it was time to change the locks and skilfully installed a Yale lock in the bedroom door. As we stood admiring her handiwork she gave it one last blow with the hammer – and shifted the doorpost away from the brick wall. This meant, of course, that the door would not close and Consuelo spent the next four hours shaving wood off the door so that we could close it. It was with immense relief that we retired to bed with our flock, secure in the knowledge that no one could raid us in our absence.

Eventually, it was time to move on and I signed up to do a three-month locum in the general practice in the Oxford suburb of Blackbird Leys. We were lucky in finding a country cottage to rent and moved our entourage there, having spent several hours returning our hospital room to some kind of normality.

Life in the country was splendid. We discovered that the garden was full of new potatoes and would dig them up by torchlight and have them for supper. The cottage was one of a pair of farm labourers' dwellings and our neighbours were a young doctor, Barney Williams, his wife Katy and their baby. The Williamses, living on only one salary, were poorer than us and I remember Barney gloomily recounting his bank manager's reply to a request for a loan to buy a car: 'Dr Williams,' he had said, 'if you were *given* a car you couldn't afford to keep it!'

Life with the animals was never dull. A teenage chipmunk escaped into the wild, to live happily, we hoped, for ever. The second gerbil, however, joined his brother in the great cage in the sky: driven to distraction by his rustling one night, I banished him to the bathroom only to find him in the morning floating like Ophelia in a watery grave. Luckily his parents were still out of the country so replacement was not yet urgent.

The real drama, however, came the day that Henrietta escaped and took refuge in Katy's kitchen next door. I was summoned by Katy's screams as she confronted Henrietta across the kitchen floor. I rushed to her rescue only to see Henrietta take refuge behind the Raeburn. With horrified visions of roast chipmunk I threw open the door of the stove and began raking the red-hot coals onto the stone floor. Katy was not amused but I was a mother possessed and refused to stop until all the fire was out on the kitchen floor. We shone a torch behind the Raeburn and revealed a terrified Henrietta who had managed to wedge herself between the stove and the wall. A Raeburn is a solid-fuel cooker built largely of cast iron and almost completely immovable. I was beside myself and insisted on going out in the car to the phone box to call the fire brigade. I can't recall what they said, but the fire brigade were not keen to come out into the country on a rainy Saturday night to rescue a chipmunk. My next call was to the RSPCA but, it being 9.00 p.m. on Saturday night, there was only an answering machine. In desperation I turned to a firm of industrial engineers who, to my delight, agreed to come to my rescue, so I returned home to wait.

In about an hour there was a knock at the door and two burly engineers entered Katy's tiny kitchen. While I stood by with a saucepan and lid they took a crowbar to poor Katy's stove and slowly levered it away from the wall. Within seconds a furious and overheated Henrietta shot out like a bullet out of a gun only to be fielded by an expert saucepan wielder (myself). In her fury she bit me hard and I yelled out an expletive which shocked even the engineers who had expected something akin to a kitten to emerge into my outstretched arms. I thanked them profusely and, having apologised to Katy yet again, went thankfully off to bed.

The story should end here, but at 8.00 a.m. on the following Sunday morning Consuelo and I were woken by an extremely officious RSPCA officer who demanded to inspect Henrietta and report upon her injuries. Rather crossly we led him to her cage where she had commenced her morning ablutions, suffering from nothing more than a set of slightly singed whiskers. At last convinced, he left us to enjoy the remains of our Sunday morning in bed.

This saga would not be complete without an account of The Great Gerbil Deception when David's friends returned to the UK to be reunited with their pets. David was not amused when we returned from Devon with news of Scrumpy's demise but he was horrified to learn that Stumpy had such an ignominious end. We were less concerned, reckoning that one gerbil must be pretty much like another. We were wrong, however, because Stumpy and Scrumpy were indeed rare gerbils and no pet shop we tried had anything larger than your ordinary run-of-the-mill, small, rat-sized gerbil. Eventually, defeated, we bought two small grey rodents and left it to David to explain to his friends how it had come about that their pets had shrunk. The morning they were due back, however, David went to inspect them only to find one very fat gerbil preening its whiskers and just enough evidence to make it abundantly clear that the other animal had not run away.

In November of 1968 tragedy struck our family when my mother was involved in a car crash in the Devon lanes. My father was driving but they had dual controls in the car and it seems that my mother put her foot under the brake pedal on her side so that when he pressed *his* pedal the brakes failed. My mother sustained a mild head injury and was hospitalised overnight. The following morning, however, while awaiting discharge she suffered a massive stroke, or, to be more medically accurate, bilateral subdural haemorrhages. She was rushed to the operating theatre, but despite surgery she never regained consciousness.

I went down to Devon to see her and found seeing her unconscious unbearably sad. I was back in Oxford, working as a GP locum, when my father phoned with news of her death. I was actually with a patient when the call came through so I could only weep briefly and return to finish my surgery. I was desperately saddened at her death for I had always loved her much more than my father and I enjoyed her company so much. In some ways, I am very like her: artistic, untidy, good with my hands and a competent but slapdash cook. We both loved poetry and, having good memories, would quote it endlessly to each other. Most of all, we shared a passion for animals, especially dogs. She always had cairn terriers but I'm sure she would have been entranced by my gloriously leonine, if disobedient, chows. Now that I am myself 67, the age at which she died, I would so love to talk to her as an equal.

Sometime in December our Oxford jobs came to an end and Consuelo and I moved to Leicester, she to a highly coveted post as registrar in plastic surgery and me to see what SHO jobs were available in the Leicester Royal Infirmary.

NOTES
1. A degloving injury involves the removal of all the skin.

9

⁂

THE MENAGERIE MOVES
TO LEICESTER:
1969

C onsuelo and I were extremely reluctant to leave Oxford but all
good things come to an end and we determined to enjoy
Leicester. With us we took Penny, the red and blue macaw,
Alexander, the small green parrot, and Henrietta, the only
surviving chipmunk. There being no suitable hospital accommodation,
we rented a flat and set up home with our family.

I decided to take any job going and soon found a vacancy in surgery
and then another in orthopaedics at the Leicester Royal Infirmary.
Eventually I got an SHO post in the Accident and Emergency
Department where we were kept busy with road-traffic accidents from
the nearby motorway and the usual run of minor injuries, which are the
bread and butter of casualty work all over the world. As in Oxford I loved
the work of mending and comforting people and was deeply content in
my new life. Consuelo, meanwhile, was working for Maurice Kinmouth,
a charming and debonair plastic surgeon who welcomed us both to his
home without asking any awkward questions.

There is no doubt that I loved Consuelo more than I have ever loved
anyone else, man or woman, but this was a love for the person she was,
not a desire for sexual intimacy. Our love was fulfilled in a sharing of life
and ideas and, of course, a common besotted devotion to our various
beasts. More than that, Consuelo had a deep vulnerability which
appealed to my own need to take care of another human being and make

a home for him or her. Consuelo's difficulty was that she was extremely shy and had learned in her teens that alcohol bolstered her courage. It took me a while to realise that her drinking was a problem, but once I did, it became my job to help her control her intake.

It was during our time at the Elizabeth Court flat that Winston, the red-gold chow-chow, came into our lives. I can't quite remember how it came about but we liberated him from a sort of puppy farm which sold many different breeds of dogs to the not too discerning customer. My passion for furry creatures overcame me and we went home with a small russet-coloured puppy who was to be my constant companion for the next six or seven years of my life. I was in seventh heaven and happily took care of his every need including taking him out to pee in the snow at three in the morning – glimpsing by chance those who were stealthily decamping by night to avoid paying their rent!

Chows, I was to learn, are very singular animals. Nominally dogs, they are said to have descended both from wolves and from bears. They have a thick coat, a very curly tail and a face which is reminiscent of a lion, framed as it is by a red-brown mane. They are seriously one-woman dogs: utterly devoted and affectionate to their owners but often wary of strangers. They are also, alas, famous for their stubborn temperament and you can consider yourself deeply honoured if they deign to come to you when called. In the country they are a major liability, their powerful hunting instinct sending them after sheep, cats, anything on four legs, but in the city they are wonderful: the perfect companion night and day for the professional man or woman. To prove my point I have a photograph of Sigmund Freud and his two chows in their home in cosmopolitan Vienna! Chow owners are completely besotted about the breed: I am frequently approached by people who are desperate to tell me that their gran or the woman next door had a chow when they were five. One woman rushed up to show me the photograph of her beloved chow, which she was still carrying in her wallet twenty years after the dog itself had died.

With hindsight I find it ironic that as a young woman I had secretly despised my mother for being so neurotic about her dogs, only to find that, after she died, whatever spirit it was entered into my soul. Now, in my retirement, I have two chows: red Anka, to anchor me to Plymouth, and black Mollie, who is a wicked xenophobe who barks furiously at any passing asylum-seeker. More (of course!) of these later.

After about a year we were given a beautiful hospital-owned apartment much nearer the centre of town. By this time we had three chows: my Winston, Consuelo's black dog Joshua and his mate Jericho. The names are taken, of course, from Holy Scripture, or rather from the Negro spiritual 'Joshua fought the battle of Jericho and the walls came tumbling down'! I should explain that having two male chows and a bitch is about the stupidest thing we ever did because, of course, when the bitch was in season the two males fought. There was one hideous occasion when I was alone in the flat, Consuelo having gone to Paris for a week, and Jericho came on heat.

With the help of the vet, I doped both male dogs, which kept them relatively quiet, but at seven o'clock one morning, I heard ferocious growling and found that Joshua had my beloved Winston by the throat and seemed determined to kill his rival. Without thinking I put my hands into Joshua's mouth and wrenched open his jaws, freeing Winston but sustaining some very nasty bites on both hands. I shut the two dogs in separate rooms and leant out of the window to cry for help. Two passing workmen came to my rescue, and seeing my hands exclaimed, 'You need a doctor!', at which I sobbed piteously, 'But I *am* a doctor!'

There was nothing for it but to take sick leave until my hands were healed, so I put Joshua into kennels and got a kind friend to drive me and the other two dogs to Devon. Just who looked after the parrots and the long-haired Peruvian guinea pigs I don't quite remember. Henrietta, alas, had come to a sticky end when we first moved to Leicester and the new flat, for with mattresses on the floor there was nowhere for her to escape from the dogs. She did, however, have a wonderful life, living free and hibernating for the winter in my desk, appropriating one drawer as a grain store, one as a loo and one as her nest. I wept copiously and had to hide myself in one of the cubicles in Casualty as I mourned her passing.

The high point of our career in animal husbandry was the night that Jericho was successfully delivered of eight puppies. Consuelo played midwife while I supervised another confinement: that of my long-haired Peruvian guinea pig. The guinea pigs, alas, were born dead but the puppies were delightful. Initially tiny and fat like grubs, they grew apace to become enchanting balls of fluff staggering about on bandy legs. Jericho was a wonderful mother and between us we managed to rear all eight: the most beautiful, a dog, Consuelo earmarked for her cousin Luz-Maria in Santiago, who named him Slangivar. The rest went to various people either for money or as gifts; I don't really remember.

Sometime in 1969, I was appointed to be in day-to-day charge of casualty, responsible for the work of eleven doctors, some junior and some GPs with an interest in emergency work. Professionally it was a wonderful time, for I loved nothing better than the multiple challenges of emergency medicine and trauma. I found the major road-traffic-accident victims and the fight to save their lives thrilling: one had to be constantly alert to changes in the patient's physical condition and level of consciousness lest he or she suddenly deteriorate with internal bleeding or an unsuspected head injury.

Once stabilised, the patients were moved to the ward or, more often, to the operating theatre, and I would return to deal with the endless queue of minor injuries, trying to be patient with those who complained about the time they had waited. It was not always easy to keep one's cool, and one particularly busy afternoon I dealt with an anxious fireman who had a barely visible laceration on his finger. Weary and exasperated beyond words, I advised him to suck it and told him that next time I had a fire in my waste-paper basket I would give him a ring. Mostly, however, I loved seeing the walking wounded and delighted in suturing their wounds.

As time went by I realised that the only way I could advance in knowledge and experience was to do more time in general surgery, and for that I needed the second part of the FRCS, the Fellowship of the Royal College of Surgeons. This was the time before Accident and Emergency medicine became a recognised speciality and I knew that I would never get a surgical registrar's job without any exams. Once again, therefore, I returned to my books and prepared to meet the examiners. I eventually sat the exam in Edinburgh in 1971 and was so sure that I'd passed that I presented myself to hear the numbers of the successful candidates read out. It was only when I realised that they had passed my number without calling it that I knew that I had failed and went sadly back to my hotel. I had done very well in the written papers but was let down by my lack of practical surgical experience when the examiner asked me about the prostatic veins.

Realising that I had been lucky to do as well as I had, I decided there was nothing for it but to get general surgical experience. That meant moving from Leicester because, I figured, I had no chance competing with the young men. My only hope, I thought, was to try for a place at a women's hospital such as the Elizabeth Garrett Anderson or the Royal Free Hospital for women. The idea of working in an all-female environment, however, filled me with gloom because I so enjoyed the companionship of the men. This was 1971 and there were far more men than women in hospital medicine and I had always enjoyed being the only girl in a team. It was with this in mind that I began to consider seriously Consuelo's idea that I should accompany her to Chile and get my 'cutting experience' there.

Life for Consuelo over the past few months had become increasingly difficult. The first thing that happened was that her international driving licence had expired and, no matter how hard she tried, she couldn't manage to pass the English driving test. Her beloved black Rover had therefore to be abandoned for a humble motor scooter and an L plate. One weekend, some Chilean friends of hers arrived in London and Consuelo took the train to meet them. Against all advice she drove to the station in the unlicensed Rover to which she had appended the scooter's up-to-date tax disc so that she could drive her friends back to the house when they returned from London.

She could so easily have got away with it but when she and her friends approached the car they found a tall policeman standing over it. I don't recall how they got the car home but I have vivid memories of us plotting what we could say in court when she was charged with driving an unlicensed vehicle. Consuelo, as I have explained, had no problem about lying and eventually concocted a story in which the tax discs had been mixed up and placed quite innocently on the wrong vehicles. I agreed to give evidence on her behalf and after I had given my version of the story the prosecuting solicitor fixed me with a beady eye and said, 'Dr Cassidy, I put it to you that you are lying to save your friend.' Not wishing to compound my felony, I exclaimed, 'But I'm on oath!' Absurdly, I can't recall the verdict but my memory is that Consuelo was fined a hundred pounds and we escaped, thankful that she had not incurred a more serious penalty.

Despite her ability to bend the truth, Consuelo was a woman of enormous integrity and during the eight years of our friendship she influenced me profoundly, opening my mind to the injustice of poverty and exploitation in the developing world. I should, of course, have learned about this at my mother's knee or at least at university, but the fact was that my parents were like most people caught up with their own problems and at Oxford I was oblivious to all but medicine and my possible call to religious life. With hindsight, Consuelo, who was a professed agnostic, if not an atheist, was infinitely more open to gospel values than I was. She had a natural empathy with the underdog and, had she not died young, might have done great things in pre- and post-coup Chile.

It is a real sadness to me, now, that Consuelo never met the friends whom I acquired after her death, for I'm sure they would have given her a very different idea of Christianity in general and Catholicism in particular. In the early days of our friendship we discussed religion frequently and, although she never tried to influence my beliefs, I slowly drifted away from the practice of Catholicism during our time together. When Consuelo died in 1974, however, I immediately sought comfort in religion again and deeply regretted the years of my 'lapsing'. With hindsight, I no longer see myself as having 'strayed' because my life was so full of love and caring both for Consuelo and my patients. I believe that my meeting and loving Consuelo was a vital part of my 'formation' as a human being and as a Christian, for without her I might have continued my life as blind to the existence of poverty and injustice as I was when we first met.

'Ubi caritas et amor, Deus ibi est', 'Where love and charity are dwelling, God is living there.' Understanding the truth of this verse from an ancient Latin hymn has been a revelation to me in later years, as has the depth and simplicity of the following passage from Micah:

> 'With what gift shall I come into Yahweh's presence
>   and bow down before God on high?
> Shall I come with holocausts,
>   with calves one year old?
> Will he be pleased with rams by the thousand,
>   with libations of oil in torrents?
> Must I give my first-born for what I have done wrong,
>   the fruit of my body for my own sin?'
> – What is good has been explained to you, man;
>   this is what Yahweh asks of you:
>   only this, to act justly,
>   to love tenderly
>   and to walk humbly with your God. (Micah 6:6–8)

As I understand it, what the prophet is saying is this: don't get carried away with religious ceremony, with cathedral liturgies, however beautiful, and don't think that you have to give up those you love because of the religious law. This is what the Lord asks of you, only this: be just and honest in your business dealings, be generous with what you have and share with those who have less. Most importantly, love your neighbour, your wife, your kids and those around you. Don't hurt them with cruel words or neglect but reveal to them that they are precious in God's eyes. 'Walk humbly with your God' speaks to me of admission of my own frailty and humanity: my jealousy, greed, meanness and all the other weaknesses of which I am ashamed.

I wish I could have shared these passages with Consuelo: she would have been amazed, for the Catholicism of her childhood was what Marx called the 'opium of the poor'. The religion which told people: 'Be good now, work hard, obey the boss, go to church every Sunday, deny your carnal urges and you will receive your reward in heaven.'

As a medical student, Consuelo had been exposed to the terrible poverty and degradation of the Santiago poor. Ill fed, ill housed and ill educated, they lived in shanty towns, drinking for solace and to escape the misery of watching their malnourished babies dying of diarrhoea and pneumonia. Realising that the only solution was a political one, Consuelo became friends with the young Communists but never had enough commitment to work with them. A rebel like her mother, she found the discipline of the party too confining.

Consuelo was a dreamer and, alas, also an alcoholic. While we lived together I was able to control the amount she drank but it was still enough to give her the cirrhosis of which she eventually died. It was during that year of 1971 that Consuelo had to have her gall bladder removed and the cirrhosis was found at surgery. The doctor looking after her told her that, unless she stopped drinking, she would be dead within a couple of years, but she kept that from me for a long time.

It was in 1971 that Dr Salvador Allende was elected as Chile's first Marxist president and Consuelo decided she must return home to be part of the new Chile. I was deeply unhappy, partly because I was enormously fond of her but also because I feared that without my influence she would drink herself to death. She was, however, adamant and resigned her job and flew to Chile with her two beloved chows, determined to contribute to the birth of the new Chile.

I had to decide then whether or not I should follow her, especially as I was not convinced that she wanted me to come. I think she feared, not without reason, that I would have difficulty adjusting to life in a new country with a different language and such a different culture. For weeks I agonised, but when I received her letter asking me to join her I had no further doubts and resigned my now permanent position as Medical Assistant in A & E. Just what my family thought of my decision to go to Chile I never asked, although I knew that my father was very disapproving because he had such high hopes that I would become a famous doctor. My mind, however, was made up and I resigned my job and booked a passage to Chile on the SS *Brandenstein*, a German cargo boat operating between Bremerhaven and the coast of South America.

10

WINSTON AND I
GO TO CHILE:
1971

I n late November of 1971 Winston and I duly set off on our great
South American adventure, travelling by car to Dover, by ferry to
Antwerp and then by German cargo boat to the port of Valparaiso,
just north of Chile's capital city of Santiago. With us we took thirty-
three pieces of hand luggage and another eleven in the hold. Finding the
cost of professional packing more than I could afford, I packed everything myself: the full-length mirror travelled between two mattresses
which I wrapped up in a carpet, while the smaller goods were packed
securely in the cage belonging to the mynah bird. The fridge I wrapped in
an eiderdown and my clothes travelled happily in their chest of drawers.
Apart from three beds, a table and a few chairs, these were to be our only
possessions for the next four years.

The journey by sea took five weeks, taking us across the Atlantic
Ocean, through the Panama Canal and down the west coast of South
America to the rather sleazy port of Buenaventura in Colombia. From
there we travelled to Guyaquil in Equador, Callao in Peru and thence
down the west coast of Chile to the port of Valparaiso. The beginning of
the journey was a nightmare as I couldn't persuade Winston to pee on the
boat. He held out for the thirty-six hours between Antwerp and
Amsterdam and another thirty-six until we arrived at Bremerhaven. After
that there was only the North Sea and the Atlantic Ocean and I feared that

he might die of pride. I can remember walking him on deck in my night-gown in icy rain and meeting a member of the crew who muttered dourly, 'Dogs die at sea!' Eventually, however, he found a very smelly pile of rope and pronounced it suitable, nearly flooding the deck as he did so.

From then on it was plain sailing. No kennel had been provided, so Winston travelled in my cabin and initially in my bunk, wedged between me and the wall as the listing of the ship meant he slid backwards and forwards across the cabin floor in a rather unsettling manner. My companion passengers on the ship were a middle-aged German woman and her teenage son, and the Peruvian wife of the first engineer who spoke neither English nor German. We dined each night with the Captain and passed the days reading or playing Scrabble with a German set. As we entered warmer waters, however, they put up a wood and canvas swimming pool and I swam happily while Winston, tied securely to the ship's railings, looked on doubtfully.

When I was neither swimming nor reading, Winston and I would sit together next to the laundry, listening to the Chinese laundryman singing as he worked. As I watched the waves sparkling in the sunlight I felt very close to God and prayed that this adventure would turn out OK. I had, in fact, good reason to pray, for I spoke not a word of Spanish and had no idea whether my English medical degree would be acceptable to the Chileans. I knew only that I wanted to be with Consuelo and the rest would have to be sorted out when I arrived.

Eventually, on 22 December, we reached the port of Valparaiso and I began to worry about getting Winston through the customs, for I had not enquired about quarantine restrictions. My next worry came with the news that it was too rough for the ship to dock and passengers would be taken ashore by launch. This meant that we would not be disembarking where expected and I wondered how we would even make contact with Consuelo. I need not have worried on the first count, however, for when Winston went for his veterinary inspection, the man patted him all over and said, 'What a lovely dog', and we were free!

So there I was, with my dog on a lead, on Chilean soil, but with no idea what to do next. We wandered round the streets and then as we passed a café, I heard someone call my name. To my amazement and delight, there was Consuelo with another woman, her cousin Luz Maria, the proud owner of our first-born chow puppy Slangivar. I don't remember the details, but we travelled back by car to Santiago and, with great pride, Consuelo showed me the house she had bought, Number 285, in the Calle Francisco Bilbao. There waiting for us were, of course, Joshua and

Jericho and also Consuelo's maid Mercedes who was to become such an integral part of our family.

If I had known that day what the next four years would bring, would I have stayed? Who knows? For then it was enough that I was reunited with Consuelo and our beloved chows. The next few weeks, however, were not easy. As I had feared, Consuelo was drinking heavily: a litre of Cuban rum a day, and whereas in the UK I had controlled her drinking, in Chile our roles were reversed and I had no power. At thirty-three, I was totally inexperienced in adapting to different cultures and found it really difficult to fit in with her friends. People were enormously kind to me but inevitably they wearied of speaking English and I felt totally excluded when they spoke in their rapid Chilean Spanish.

Absurdly, one of the hardest things to adapt to was the difference in meal times. We would go out to dinner with friends at around eight but dinner was rarely served until 10 p.m. or later, by which time I was desperate with hunger. Everyone else was happy drinking the Chilean national drink of Pisco Sour while I, who get tipsy after one small sherry, sat there miserably longing for my supper.

Consuelo, of course, wanted to show me off as her English friend and became exasperated that I was such a social misfit. Quite soon after my arrival it was decided that I must have intensive Spanish lessons and Consuelo's friend Jaime (not his real name) came daily to the house to teach me. Jaime was a delight: an exceptionally gentle man with a wonderful sense of humour and endless patience with my stumbling efforts to speak his language.

In the March of 1972 something happened to change my life and my relationship with Consuelo for ever and plunged me into a state of misery the like of which I have never experienced before or since.

Consuelo received a telephone call from 'Jessica', a friend we had known in Oxford, who announced that she was coming to stay for a month – or was it three? – in order to study for some exams. From the time she arrived, things were very different and I hardly ever saw Consuelo alone again. Jessica was somehow always there and I felt increasingly excluded.

Relationship difficulties are so humiliating, and yet I suspect they are the cause of the greatest suffering we humans endure. I was lonely and hurt and jealous, not to mention stony broke and utterly miserable in a foreign country. I tried to talk to Consuelo but she told me not to be stupid, and as time went by I became increasingly depressed. My salvation came when friends of Consuelo persuaded Hernan Ruiz, an

English-speaking cardiologist at the nearby San Borja hospital, to let me join his team in an honorary capacity.

From that time on, my life improved enormously, for not only did I have something useful to do but I had a new friend in Greta, a young German doctor whose husband was working in Chile for a pharmaceutical company. She was also attached to the cardiology team and we immediately became the best of friends. Greta would invite me to her home and on outings with her husband Dierk, and we had wonderful picnics in the beautiful countryside surrounding the city. My great embarrassment, however, was that I was unable to return their hospitality and invite them back to the house for fear of finding Consuelo drunk. By now she was drinking steadily throughout the day and, though she still managed to hold down her job, I never knew when an extra drink would tip her over into intoxication.

Despite my sadness at home, I was starting to find my feet. I would go twice a week to the open-air market to buy vegetables and the wonderful shellfish for which Chile is famous. There were *locos*: a tough and strong-tasting shellfish which is, I think, the same as *abalone*, *machas* and *almejas*, not unlike mussels. Mercedes taught me to make loco soup and insisted, too, that I develop a taste for *erizos*, the sea urchins which are such a prized delicacy. More to my taste was *pastel de choclo*, a wonderful dish of sweetcorn and mincemeat, and *humitas*, little parcels of corn puree wrapped up in the leaves of the corn cobs. The greatest delicacy for all Chileans, however, is beans, especially the *porotos nuevos*, the new young beans at the start of the season. Alas, philistine that I was, I longed for Heinz Baked Beans, and worried dreadfully about the wind the Chilean beans gave me.

At the hospital, my life was improving in leaps and bounds as my grasp of Spanish improved and I accepted that Chilean medicine was very different from its UK equivalent. The pattern of disease itself was different, largely I think because of the social structure of the country. In Chile, as in the rest of Latin America, 90 per cent of the land and wealth was in the hands of about 4 per cent of the populace. The middle class were comfortably off but the poor were very poor indeed. The children, in particular, suffered from the inadequate housing and indifferent diet of the urban poor, so that malnutrition, diarrhoea and chest infections were commonplace. Among the adult population there was a far higher incidence of valvular heart disease because of inadequately treated streptococcal infections, which led to damage to the heart valves.

Sometime in 1972 I was given a job as resident doctor on the coronary care unit. Even thinking about it makes me nervous now as cardiology has never been my forte. The unit was staffed by university-trained nurses who were highly skilled, and between us we managed to keep the patients alive. I did, however, achieve one minor triumph which greatly increased my standing in the department. The case was that of a young man with severe cardiac failure who was admitted for terminal care. While one of the junior cardiologists and I were looking at his chest X-ray I suddenly noticed a series of small notches on his upper ribs. Although I had never seen this before I knew their significance and exclaimed with delight, 'He's got a co-arctation of the aorta!' He did indeed have this rare condition in which a congenital narrowing of the aorta leads to the development of a collateral circulation system which by-passes the obstruction. It is these extra blood vessels which run over the ribs and, by pressure, cause the notch formation. The joy of this condition is that it can be corrected by surgery to the aorta, so by making this diagnosis I was opening up the possibility of cure for the patient.

You may wonder why this hadn't been diagnosed years earlier; I have no answer, save that I was lucky that day, largely because, as a doctor trained in trauma diagnosis, I always looked carefully at the ribs for fractures while the cardiologists instinctively looked at the heart shadow to make their diagnoses.

As time went on and it seemed likely that I would stay in Chile, I applied for permission to work as a doctor and found that I must spend a year doing attachments in the main specialities and take an exam in each. My friends, the cardiologists, signed me up for the medical place-ment, announcing that they would waive the exam because of my diagnostic success. My next placement was in surgery under the super-vision of a delightful woman surgeon, Dr Rosita Fagre, who kindly introduced me to a rich and successful plastic surgeon who paid me to assist him as he operated on his private patients. One weekend he invited me to visit him at his home in the south of Chile where I got a taste of how the really wealthy Chileans lived.

Although my Spanish was improving daily I still made some embar-rassing mistakes, particularly in using the rather vulgar language of my friendly workmen. My most memorable mistake occurred one sultry afternoon while I was talking to a middle-aged woman with varicose veins in a very large open ward. Intending to enquire whether or not her varicose eczema itched (*picazon*), I enquired, '*Senora, tiene pico?*', which translates roughly as 'Lady, do you have a willy?' The other women in the ward who had been listening with fascination to my stumbling interrogation collapsed in shrieks of laughter and I made a whole new group of friends.

After I had completed my three months in surgery I did a placement in obstetrics and gynaecology. My only memory of this is a sad one for it is of the day I was shown a ward of fifty women all of whom were yellow with jaundice caused by septicaemia from the bacterium Clostridium perfringens, a bug which thrives in deep wounds that the air cannot get to. These were all women who had had backstreet abortions provoked by inserting a stick of *perejil*, or parsley into the womb. My memory is that I was told that the majority of these women would die of their infection.

My next placement was in paediatrics and I was sent to work in a children's hospital on the outskirts of the city. Here I came face to face with the abject poverty which lay at the heart of the Chilean 'revolution'. There were under-nourished babies bottle-fed on water, dehydrated babies with diarrhoea, and feverish babies with all manner of infections. These families lived in wooden shacks in the shanty towns, often without running water or toilet. I remember learning in public health that 25 per cent of Chilean homes at that time had no lavatory of any kind: not even a chemical toilet. It is this co-existence of squalid poverty and cultured living that is so shocking in the developing world and it is no coincidence that Allende and many of his supporters were doctors. After the coup I learned that the cardiology unit at the San Borja Hospital, which took me so warmly to its heart, consisted largely of supporters of Allende's government, and a number of them were members of an elite group know as the GAP, the personal guards of the president. It was during these months at the San Borja that I became increasingly aware of the tension between Allende's followers and the 'Momios': the 'Mummies' who were against his socialist revolution. Men and women who had hitherto joked about their political differences began to avoid each other or talk angrily behind their colleagues' backs.

While I was doing my placement at the Roberto del Rio children's hospital, Chile experienced its first medical strike in which pro- and anti-Allende doctors who had hitherto worked together became irrevocably divided. My friends at the San Borja continued working, covering for their right-wing colleagues, but at the Roberto del Rio things were very different because most of the doctors were against Allende and desperate to bring about his downfall. At the height of the strike I was left with a young Russian woman doctor to care for a ward full of desperately ill babies. When one baby gave up its struggle for life we gave mouth-to-mouth respiration in a desperate effort to resuscitate it. Our efforts, however, were to no avail, for the baby died, and the doctor in charge reprimanded us and made us rinse out our mouths with 100 per cent alcohol to sterilise any germs we might have acquired.

As time passed, political tensions rose and I was suspended from my placement at the Roberto del Rio, as were all foreign nationals, because it was assumed we were Allende supporters. Our lives at home became increasingly difficult because of the lorry drivers' strike, which eventually precipitated the military coup. The strike (funded by the CIA who paid the lorry drivers US$5 a day to strike) meant that many staple foods and goods were in short supply or simply unavailable. Rice, cooking oil, spaghetti, sugar and coffee all disappeared from the shops. I have a vivid memory of the empty shelf where the spaghetti used to be in our corner shop and my panic that I would have nothing on which to feed the dogs. This must have been just a few days before the military coup, which happened on 11 September 1973 and was to bring a bloody end to Chile's proud record of one hundred years of democracy.

11

THE DEATH OF DEMOCRACY IN CHILE: SEPTEMBER 1973

The city was strangely quiet that night of 10 September, the eve of the Generals' coup. The streets were empty as Consuelo and I returned home from visiting a neighbour, but then we had no intimation about what was to befall this lovely country. We had been engaged in the desperate act of helping to put down one of a family of seventeen cats belonging to an elderly woman who could no longer afford to feed her pets and had no money to pay the vet to do the lethal act.

On the morning of the coup I went to the *feria*, the outdoor market, to buy fruit and vegetables and anything else available. While I was there planes came overhead and we realised that they were bombing the city centre: in fact it was the Moneda, the house of government, where Allende and his men were working.

Shoppers and stallholders alike panicked and the market was rapidly evacuated. I grabbed a handful of greens from a deserted stall and made my way home as quickly as I could. I arrived home to find Consuelo listening to the radio from which issued the harsh voices of the military announcing that Allende had been overthrown and that Chile now had a military government.

As the day passed they broadcast a list of names of men and women who were to present themselves to the authorities. Among these was

Victor Jara, the famous guitar singer who died at the hands of the military during the first few days of the coup.

Consuelo was desperately worried about her sisters, one of whom worked closely with Carlos Altimarano, the head of the Communist party. Carmen arrived at our house the following day having walked miles from the factory where she was working. During these first few days there was a 24-hour curfew and we watched in disbelief as trucks of armed soldiers with their rifles pointing at us passed by our house. Even more unnerving were the limousines containing senior military personnel that flashed past us at all hours of the day and night.

After a few days, the 24-hour curfew was lifted and we were allowed out until four, then six o'clock in the evening. On the first possible day I went to the local supermarket and was amazed to find the shelves crammed with food that we had not seen for months: chicken, beef, fish, flour, oil, rice and spaghetti – all the staple foods that had been withdrawn in order to provoke discontent and anxiety among the people. There was, however, a new problem: the price, for the goods were now way beyond most ordinary people's budget. A few days later, they were still there, the chickens cut into segments and beginning to smell because no one had the money to buy them.

These were frightening days and we stayed mainly at home, wondering if we would be visited by the military. Consuelo soon returned to work at the Posta but it was some time before I was able to resume the hospital attachments which were vital for my registration as a doctor in Chile.

By October it became apparent that Consuelo was ill with cirrhosis and Jessica and I worried about her failing health. By Christmas she was unable to work and we spent our days quietly at home, worrying about the fate of those in the hands of the secret police. Both Consuelo's sisters went into exile, Marie-Elena and her family to Canada and Carmen to Equador. We heard news of the repression from visiting friends and also from the local pharmacist who spoke of interrogation with torture and execution by firing squad in both of the city sports stadia.

Little by little we adapted to life under the military dictatorship, keeping our mouths shut in public places and scurrying home with other commuters in time for the nightly curfew. Minutes after it fell, the streets, now empty of people, would be full of cars carrying senior military personnel to who knows what meetings. Then came the army lorries full of armed military on their way to seek out anyone whom they felt was a threat to the new regime. People were constantly picked up for interrogation, usually with torture, and held while any information they had revealed was acted upon. When no longer of use they were released or simply 'disappeared', never to be seen again. At night, a helicopter without lights would circle over the city and we trembled when the occasional shot rang out in a nearby street.

Christmas came and went with no real rejoicing. At new year the silence of the curfew was broken by a lone trumpeter playing the last post: an eerie tribute to the imprisoned and the dead. By January, Consuelo's condition was worse, but it never occurred to me that she would die. At the end of February, however, she agreed to go into hospital and, on 4 March 1974, Consuelo died of liver failure. She was in her early forties: too young by far to die.

When Consuelo was admitted to hospital she was removed from the comforting alcohol which was her downfall. Once sober, she was a different woman: the old Consuelo whom I had loved and admired so much. At last we were able to talk openly again and it was as if the misunderstandings of the past months had never been. Reassured, I threw myself into trying to care for her, bringing in fruit juice to try and tempt her to drink. On 4 March, however, she began to haemorrhage; I offered my blood to transfuse her but she died before it could be given. Unable to believe that she had gone, I left the hospital in a daze and returned home to tell Mercedes of her beloved Consuelo's death.

Jessica and I were both devastated but somehow unable to comfort each other. I wanted nothing more than for her to leave, but Consuelo, who had made a will shortly before she died, had left the house to both of us, so I struggled to behave in a civilised manner.

Within days of Consuelo's death, a new friend entered our lives. Pancha, short for Francisca, was Consuelo's cousin and she came to offer her help with the funeral arrangements. Oh, how I wish I'd known Pancha while Consuelo was still alive: she was a delightful, warm-hearted and intelligent mother of eight who helped me to recover my sense of proportion. Although I was desperately sad at Consuelo's death, I realised that she had been mercifully spared seeing her beloved Chile ravaged by the military dictatorship. Despite my sadness, I was aware of a profound change in myself, a breaking of the chains which had held me bound for nearly eight years. Now I was free to be myself once more: to decide where I would live my life and with whom.

Not long after the funeral, Pancha asked if she and her three younger children could move in with Jessica and myself in the Bilbao house. Jessica and I were both delighted and soon the house, which had seemed so bleak and empty, rang with the sound of music and laughter. Pancha's family consisted of Juanito and Francisca, both in their teens, and four-year-old Carlitos, the love child of Pancha's new relationship with Argentinean-born film-maker Carlos.

Eventually my life returned to a degree of normality and I was able to continue my hospital placements in the four key specialties of medicine, surgery, obstetrics and paediatrics. I must have finished these by June or July and I spent the next few weeks trudging from office to office for the various certificates and signatures which were required for my recognition as a doctor.

Jessica's situation, of course, was very different from my own for she had not learned Spanish and had never had any real intention of working in Chile. She was, however, very depressed after Consuelo's death and spent many hours talking to Pancha. After three or four months, she decided to return to the UK and both Pancha and I helped her to sort out her clothes and the things she needed to return home. The house, as I have mentioned, belonged to both of us but I was able to buy Jessica's share with money left to me by Consuelo. All these negotiations took time but Pancha supported us both and at last the day came when Jessica was able to say goodbye to Chile and look forward to resuming her life in England. Her departure marked the close of one of the most painful chapters of my life, but also the beginning of something new and amazing which was to set me in a direction I had never dreamed of.

When Consuelo died I returned quite instinctively to the practice of my faith. Although I had not been to church for several years I started to attend Mass daily and prayed to know what I should do. To my surprise and chagrin I began to wonder once more if I was being called to enter religious life. I still had no *desire* to be a nun but the thought haunted me and intruded cruelly upon my new-found sense of happiness and freedom.

Pancha, although from the same social background as Consuelo, had retained her religious faith and had many friends among Santiago's Christian Left. Among these were the two Roberts: Father Robert Plasker, in his fifties, and Bob Neidhardt, a much younger priest. Both men belonged to the Holy Cross congregation which runs the well-known American University of Notre Dame, and lived in a shanty town on the northern foothills of the city. I liked them both enormously and drank in all they had to say about working with the poor and the oppressed.

This was the first time I had met anyone belonging to the radical Latin

American church and my heart burned within me as they spoke of how they tried to live the gospel message instead of just preaching it. After we had met a couple of times they invited me to visit them and have a meal. When I went I couldn't believe what I saw, for here were middle-class, educated men living in something resembling a large garden shed. The most powerful moment for me, however, was when I was asked to fetch a chair from Bob Neidhardt's room and found that all he possessed (or so it seemed to me) was a shirt and a spare pair of jeans hung on a nail on the bedroom door. From that moment on, I knew that I wanted to be part of this group of 'stripped down' people who had dared to take the gospel message seriously; I decided to stay in Chile instead of returning to the UK.

Once I had my Chilean medical qualifications I was ready to begin my new life but decided that I would visit my family in England before I settled down to work. My father had sent me an open ticket to the UK soon after the coup, so all I had to do was book my flight, secure in the knowledge that Pancha and Mercedes would look after my dogs and the house. In August of 1974 I flew with British Caledonian Airways to London's Heathrow and took the train for Devon.

12

INTERLUDE IN ENGLAND:
1974

I arrived back in Devon in August to find my father on the verge of being hospitalised for colon cancer. When I look back upon this time I realise how badly I handled his illness. We visited him in hospital, of course, but I have no recollection of talking to him about his illness and its possible outcome.

It was a joy to be back with my brother and his wife and we delighted in our usual summer pursuits of walking down the estuary at low tide and picnicking on the beach. But my heart was in Chile with Pancha and my dogs and I longed to return and begin my new life as part of a radical Christian Church. My hopes, however, were rudely dashed by the news that my house had been raided by the secret police and Pancha and her husband Carlos taken prisoner. I was told by friends that the DINA, the secret police, believed that I was in Europe collecting money for the Chilean resistance, so it would be dangerous for me to return. I was devastated: separated from my friends and my dogs with no idea of what the future would bring.

In search of spiritual comfort, I went to London to talk to Michael Hollings, but he gave me short shrift because I talked endlessly about Chile and ignored the poor and dispossessed under my nose in his house. I can see now that I must have been very tiresome, but it was the first time that Michael had been sharp with me and I was very hurt. On his advice I sought out a woman called Susie Younger who had founded a lay institute of religious women. Susie was an amazing woman who had worked as a lay missionary in Korea and I liked and admired her enormously. When I went to visit her community, the Auxiliaries of the Apostolate, in Lourdes, however, I did not feel at home and longed to be back with my Chilean and North American friends.

Lourdes, nevertheless, was the setting for an enormously powerful experience of the Divine which confirmed for me that I must continue in my search for God's will for me. Lourdes, where the Blessed Virgin is said to have appeared to the young peasant girl, Bernadette Soubirous, is centred on the grotto where the apparitions took place. Beside the grotto runs the river Gave and it was here that I made a firm, if unfocused, commitment to follow Christ, for when the bell for the angelus tolled I found myself praying the words of Mary in the Magnificat, 'Be it done unto me according to thy word.'

It's strange how a familiar phrase can suddenly stand out from a hymn or poem so that one recites it as if for the first time. I stood there by the river inviting God to do whatever he wanted with me, never dreaming that he would take me up on my offer. Prayer of this kind is a bit like texting someone far away: you tap in your words – 'help!' or 'thank you!' or 'I love you!' – but you never really know that your message has been received. That night, however, I received confirmation of my message in a way that I had never dreamed.

It was the custom of the Auxiliaries of the Apostolate, with whom I was staying, to spend an hour each day before the Blessed Sacrament in prayer and I chose to 'watch' between ten and eleven o'clock in the evening. I was alone in their large chapel and the minutes dragged by, second by tedious second. People not experienced in prayer have no conception, I suspect, of how boring prayer time can be. Wordless prayer, simple waste-of-time prayer, can be sweet beyond belief but mostly one's mind is invaded by irrelevant thoughts about the day's chores or what one is going to make for dinner. Sitting there in that bleak chapel, my back ached and my nose itched and I wriggled about and looked endlessly at my watch. At last it was five to eleven, then four and then, at long last, the big hand of my watch was on the twelve and I rose thankfully to my feet and made for the door. Beyond the chapel door was the usual vestibule with a large holy water font. Cradle Catholic that I was, I dipped my right hand in the water and crossed myself – and then something very odd happened: I heard within myself the words of Jesus in the garden of Gethsemane, 'Will you not watch one hour with me?' I was not amused and muttered to the 'voice', 'But I've just spent an hour watching and I'm tired and fed up and I want to go to bed.' The 'voice', however, persisted and somehow

I knew that I had to obey, so, with extremely ill grace, I flounced back into the chapel and plonked myself back on my seat. I must stress that I was distinctly put out about the whole thing and experienced no warm feelings of devotion whatsoever. Then 'it', whatever 'it' was, hit me and I felt an overpowering sense of awe and joy as if in the presence of God. I saw nothing and I heard nothing but I felt totally overwhelmed and not a little afraid. I slid to my knees and stayed there, transfixed until, after minutes, the feeling passed and I felt completely drained. There was no further request, no message of love, just a feeling that the Lord had been in this place and the only appropriate thing was to stay quietly there.

Eventually, I returned to my room and lay for a while prostrate on the cool tiles of the bathroom floor, feeling that this was the only position in which to worship the God that I had just met.

When I returned to London I told Michael about what had happened that night and he responded briefly that my experience was genuine but I should never try to *make* it happen again. Back in Devon, my father was convalescent and frail and my brother arranged for a local woman to look after him in his own home. In November he deteriorated markedly and on 8 December he died peacefully in his own home.

I cannot pretend that I mourned his passing for, although I adored him as a child, his unspoken demands lay heavily upon me in my adult years. I always felt that he disapproved of my Chilean adventure and longed for me to make good in the British hospital system. Politically we were poles apart and my new-found socialist beliefs were alien to him. We buried him next to my mother in our local churchyard and I felt a great sense of freedom.

Christmas came and went. We gathered our remaining family about us: my brother Mike, his wife Pat and their two children Lucinda and Peter. My mother's youngest brother, Edmund, and his wife Elizabeth joined us but somehow I longed for my other, Chilean, family and felt ill at ease as we raised our glasses in the toasts to Queen and country, old friends and new relations.

After Christmas the word came through from Chile that Pancha and Carlos had been released into exile in Argentina and the DINA were no longer interested in my house in the Calle Bilbao. Desperate to return, I booked my flight and bid goodbye to my English family and set off for Latin America, via Toronto where Manena, Consuelo's sister, had gone into exile with her doctor husband and their children.

I was really looking forward to seeing Manena, as she was known, but the visit was not a success and I left with a slightly bitter taste in my mouth because it became very clear to me that Consuelo's sisters felt that her estate should have come to them. In particular, she expected me to give money to her sister Carmen and I don't think she believed me when I said I had none.

Next stop was Ecuador where I was to stay in Quito with British friends whom I had met in Chile after Consuelo died. We did a little sightseeing and I marvelled at the gilt-decorated churches and the gruesome blood-encrusted statues of Christ and his saints. I decided not to meet up with Consuelo's sister Carmen because Manena had said she was desperate for money and I didn't feel up to explaining that I had none and that Consuelo's house was now my home.

After Ecuador, I flew to Lima in Peru from whence I took the train up the mountains to the old and beautiful town of Cuzco and from there to the famous Inca ruins of Macchu Piccu. From there I made my way to the Altiplano and Lake Titicaca where I stayed in a small boarding house. My first evening was a complete nightmare because I was stricken with vomiting and diarrhoea and had to make endless trips to the lavatory anxiously clutching my passport and travellers' cheques.

The following day I made contact with some American missionaries who were working with the local people and met, by chance, another traveller. David, as I shall call him, was an American missionary priest who was taking a break between Latin American postings. I told him my story and he told me his as we sat on the banks of Lake Titicaca and watched the llamas and the famous boats made of straw. We were both suffering from the effects of altitude, nausea and shortness of breath on any exertion, and decided it was time we moved on. David was on his way to Ariquipa, the second city of Peru, and I decided to go with him.

We travelled together on the train and held hands under my poncho as we watched one of the local people tenderly caring for his little boy. Although really pleased to be back in Latin America, I was quite lonely and I was pleased to have found a friend. On arrival in Ariquipa, David helped me find a hotel and I settled in while he went to check in with the priests with whom he was staying.

Later that evening we went out to dinner, enjoying our restored vitality at the lower altitude. After we had eaten and wandered around, 'David' walked me back to my hotel and I, naive as ever, invited him up for coffee. What had I expected? Perhaps a happy prolongation of the evening with spiritual conversation: I don't know. Clearly, however, we had misread each other's signals and I was taken quite unawares when David began removing his belt. Oh, I could have said 'No. no. This is wrong,' but I didn't. I was lonely and yearning to be loved, so I gave in, as women do in all walks of life.

With hindsight, it seems that we spent the next two days in bed together, each taking time out from God and vows. As I lay in bed I looked up at the ceiling, which was laced with narrow batons. At each junction I saw a cross and told God that I was sorry, that this was a vacation, a momentary lapse, and that I would return to him as soon as I could.

What, I wonder, does God make of this kind of lapse? Who knows? The Catholic Church has always been deeply disapproving of the sins of the flesh, though illogically lenient about cruelty and denigration. I listened today to a man in his fifties describe how the nun who taught him in primary school would hook her walking stick around his neck. As Jesus said so long ago, 'Let him who is without sin cast the first stone!' I shall always have happy memories of Arequipa, with its houses and churches of white volcanic rock. I remember visiting one church with David, my heart turning over as I listened to the sound of a man singing unaccompanied, his voice like honey in the stillness of the afternoon.

After two days, our holiday was over and David and I parted to go our separate ways. My next port of call was the small Peruvian town of Chimbote, trapped between the desert and the sea, where the two Roberts were working. Both men had been expelled from Chile by the DINA for harbouring people on the run and they now worked in an even poorer place with even more desperate people. Bob Neidhardt, I remember, was about to take his final vows and we walked and talked in the dusty street, catching up with each other's news. After a few days I returned to Lima and flew across the Andes to Argentina and the beautiful city of Buenos Aires to visit Pancha. She and Carlos had been held a month by the DINA and then expelled from the country. Pancha was sad, missing her friends and her grown-up children, but put on a brave face as she showed me the sights of BA. It was so good to see her again and I was glad to bring her greetings from the two Robertos, her companions in crime in the sheltering of fugitives.

At last, the time came for me to leave and I set off, in great trepidation, for Chile. I had been told that the immigration officials had a list of all undesirables and I thought that I might well be on it. I need not have worried, however, because I passed through without difficulty and was met by a doctor friend of Consuelo's and taken home to the Calle Bilbao.

It was a strange homecoming: delightful in that I received a rapturous welcome from Mercedes and the dogs, but also scary for I knew that I was

taking a considerable risk in returning to a house now marked by the
DINA. When I look back now, I am amazed at my own courage and
determination though I suspect that, had it not been for the dogs pulling
at my heart strings, I might have found my vocation elsewhere.

13

RETURN TO CHILE:
1975

O nce back in the Bilbao house, I knew I'd come home. Mercedes, who had been Consuelo's maid long before I arrived, had banished the chows to the garden but I would have none of it and soon they were back in their rightful place on the divans which served as sofas in our house. My first priority was to get a job and I set out to find Consuelo's old boss Dr Juan Rolle, who worked at the Posta Tres, the third of Santiago's emergency hospitals. I was lucky to get a job on one of the shifts and soon settled down to my new life.

After a few weeks, I had cause to wonder if I was pregnant. Realising that 'David' was wedded to his vows, I made no attempt to contact him and told only Mercedes who was thrilled at the thought of a baby. After another two weeks, I realised that I was not pregnant, my fantasies of motherhood came to a natural end and I reordered my dreams.

Mercedes and I became good friends, united by our love of Consuelo and the dogs. By now I was reasonably fluent in Spanish and we communicated well. I set about improving my house and felt I was doing my bit for the poor by employing a *maestro chasquero*, a man of all works who is master of none. Desperate not to lose my rekindled life of prayer, I went each week on the day after the night shift to visit the Benedictine Monastery of Las Condes. Here I prayed with the monks and, when the chapel was shut, sat on a low wall gazing at the Andes mountains, which surrounded the city, as they came and went in the mist. I went each day to Mass in the Italian church around the corner but when I tried to go to confession the priest told me it would be better to seek out some Irish missionary fathers who lived not far from my house.

My first meeting with the Columbans, who lived literally round the corner, was on 18 March, the day after the feast of St Patrick. They welcomed me warmly and fed me with green ice cream: the first of many kindnesses. Our friendship was to cost them dear when, nine months later, I was arrested in their house; but that story must wait.

My next encounter with Santiago's missionary community was with an American nun, Sister Rebecca Quinn, whom I met swimming in a public pool. Rebecca was a gentle woman in her fifties who had spent most of her religious life working in Chile as a member of the American Maryknoll sisters. She invited me to her home and we spent many happy hours together drinking tea or sitting in the sun. One day, Rebecca introduced me to two younger members of her community, Ita Ford and Carla Piette, with whom I felt an instant bond, for they spoke the same faith language as the two Roberts and I was immediately warmed by their fire.

I went by bus to visit them where they lived at the end of the tracks in a *poblacion* (shanty town). Theirs was a small wooden house planted in the midst of the local community and I both admired and feared their commitment to living 'in solidarity' with the poor. I was happier when they came to visit me in my house, and as we prayed together I asked God to free me of my attachment to my rich life and my dogs. Did I really mean it? Probably not, for my dogs were my family and I could never have left them of my own free will. Little did I know that God would answer these careless prayers; but more of this later.

Through the Maryknoll sisters I met other American missionaries: Jane Kenrick, Connie Kelly, Liz Gilmore and more. It was while I was browsing through Liz's books that I came across a copy of the writings of St John of the Cross and I asked her if I could borrow it. Realising that I was not ready to digest such heavy mystical theology, Liz suggested I seek out an English Jesuit, Father Chris Wall and ask him for spiritual direction.

This is how I came one morning to be knocking nervously on the door of the Jesuit house in downtown Santiago. I'm not sure what I was expecting: probably a man in his fifties, so I was quite unprepared to be greeted by a tall, handsome Englishman of around my own age of thirty-six. Brian, known in Chile as 'Chris', Wall was a very spiritual young man with a lovely sense of humour. He listened carefully as I told him of my sense of calling to religious life and clearly took it very seriously. After an hour or so I emerged into the street completely wrung out but glad to have, at last, a companion in my search. I saw Chris a few more times until he declared firmly that he could do nothing more with me until I made a retreat, so I took a week off work and went by bus to a convent in Malloco on the outskirts of Santiago.

As a Catholic I had made retreats before but had no experience of the Spiritual Exercises of St Ignatius of Loyola, the fourteenth-century founder of the Society of Jesus, more commonly known as the Jesuits. The Exercises are a psycho-spiritual method of helping a person face herself and her maker. They are especially useful for helping individuals discern which way of life is appropriate for them personally. Over the following week I saw Chris twice a day to discuss how I felt I was being led. In his absence, I read passages of Scripture, which he chose for me, and the rest of the time I spent in prayer or alone with my own thoughts.

As the week passed it became abundantly clear to me that I felt called – and I wished – to spend my life dedicated to the service of God. From the outset I was entranced by St Ignatius's 'Principle and Foundation' at the beginning of his little book *The Spiritual Exercises*: '*El hombre es creado a alabar y servir Dios, Nuestro Senor. Todos los otros cosas sobre la haz de la tierra son para el hombre para ayudarlo conseguir a su fin.*' In English, this reads: 'Man is created to praise and serve our Lord God, thereby saving his soul. All the other things on the face of the earth are for man to help him attain the end for which he was created.' It was so clear: we are created to worship and serve God, and everything else in the world is there to help us. Ignatius continued: '*De donde se sigue que el hombre debe usar las cosas en tanto le ayude y debe quitar los in cuanto le impede consiguir a su fin.*' 'From this it follows that man must use the things of the earth in so far as they help him and must leave them in so far as they impede him from achieving his end.' It is the amazing wisdom and freedom of the '*tanto y cuanto*' which appeals to me: if a glass of red wine relaxes you and is good for your heart, great. If it makes you drunk and tiresome, then leave it alone.

Towards the end of the week, Chris gave me a passage from the book of Samuel to read: 1 Samuel 3:1, the call of Samuel. The story goes that the boy Samuel was looking after the elderly priest, Eli. One day, when Eli was taking a nap, Samuel was keeping watch in the sanctuary of the Lord. Samuel heard his name called and, thinking it was his master, went back to Eli, who said he hadn't called him. This happened again and then once more, and Eli realised it must be the Lord Yahweh who was calling the boy, so he said to him, 'Go and lie down, and if someone calls you say "Speak, Yahweh, your servant is listening". If this sounds easy, think again. If you make a genuine offer you are at grave risk of having it accepted. My favourite text among the Old Testament call narratives is the story of the prophet Isaiah who describes his sense of terrified awe in the sanctuary: he 'saw' the Lord on a high throne, surrounded by angels. 'The foundations of the threshold shook with the voice of the one who cried out, and the temple was filled with smoke.' Isaiah bemoans his unworthiness before the Lord and his lips are cleansed with burning coals. It is only then that he hears the voice of the Lord calling out: 'Whom shall I send? Who will be our messenger?' Unable to resist, Isaiah responds, 'Here I am, send me.'

That day in Malloco, I lay on a pile of dried leaves in the garden and offered myself as messenger, servant, whatever was needed. This was not a sweet religious experience but quite a violent one in which, weeping copiously, I said 'OK, damn you'.

It is as well to explain here that I never *wanted* to be a nun. I wanted to be a doctor, to get married to a man who loved me, have an exciting job, lots of dogs and a house with a swimming pool. Although I knew many nuns who were great people and seemed very happy, they lived in dreary houses populated entirely by women. It was not my idea of fun. My acceptance of what I saw as a call to religious life was an act, therefore, of foolish generosity, but at the time it brought me great spiritual and emotional peace. Chris clearly thought this was a sound decision for he encouraged me to write to the Provincial (head) of the Society of the Sacred Heart requesting admission as a novice.

The letter duly dispatched, I returned to my work at the Posta Tres to see what living with my decision did to me. The Ignatian discernment process is a wise one: you live with your newly made decision for a while before taking any irrevocable steps. If you become anxious and miserable, you think again, but if you are increasingly happy, your skin glows and your hair shines, then the chances are that your decision was a good one.

Looking back, I often wonder what was going on in the hidden reaches of my psyche that I felt so tortured by the call to be a nun. Where did the call come from? Was it truly of God or was it a product of childhood and school conditioning? The key question is, of course, do we believe that God calls people anyway?

Here my answer is a guarded 'yes': I do believe that some people experience an inner movement of the spirit in which they feel drawn or even obliged to take a particular course of action. I have no doubt that my primary call was to medicine and, with hindsight, it was nonsense to consider giving it up. What I interpreted as a call to abandon my career to follow Christ was, I believe, a culturally determined misunderstanding of a call to a close relationship with God.

I find the subject of call fascinating and delight in exploring the subject in the lives of others. My favourite, I think, is the story of Gladys Aylward, a London parlour maid in about 1910 who felt an enormously powerful call to be a missionary in China. I could quote so many other fools for Christ: Jean Vanier, the aristocratic French Canadian who has given his life to the call of people with learning difficulties, or Thérèse of Lisieux, the stubborn French fifteen-year-old who insisted upon following her sisters into an enclosed Carmelite convent and died in her twenties of consumption.

Part of my fascination with these call stories lies in the fact that I see them as the great *theophany* of our time: the shining forth or manifestation of God in our midst. This makes the scandals associated with the priesthood and the religious life all the more saddening and perplexing because priests and religious usually start their training as enthusiastic, God-centred, young people who hope to bring faith and hope to a world in which doubt and despair are endemic. What it is that snuffs out the flame in these young idealists is one of the vital questions in the Christian Church today and one which has yet to be adequately tackled.

I found myself particularly angered by what I learned from June Golding's book *The Light in the Window* (Poolbeg Press, 1998), which tells the story of 'the Magdalenes', the young illegitimately pregnant Irish girls sent by their families to be looked after by 'the good sisters' who were in reality a group of cruel, judgemental women who denigrated and exploited those in their charge. Theirs was not the terrible sin of sexual abuse (although abuse by priests did occur) but a cold-blooded lack of empathy which led to much misery and heartbreak. From the few conversations I have had on the subject with Catholic priests and nuns, the deformation of personality seems to have been a ghastly end product of attempts to 'form' the candidate as a religious. Writer Karen Armstrong's account of her own training as a novice,[1] and the impact it had upon her, is a chilling description of psychological abuse and its consequences. I count myself extremely lucky to have emerged unscathed from my eighteen-month sojourn in a convent at the age of forty.

It is important to say, before I resume my story, that not all men and women have been irrevocably damaged by harsh formation and I have many friends, both priests and nuns, who are whole, compassionate people. I thank God for their friendship and inspiration over the years.

I have greatly enjoyed exploring the theme of call or 'vocation' in the Bible and have formulated what I like to call my 'Theology of Rainbows': a simple understanding of the phenomenon which moves people to leave home and country at what they understand to be the behest of the Divine. The first call story is that of the patriarch Abraham to whom God said, quite simply, 'Go! To a place that I shall show you.'[2] This, if you think about it, is the call we all receive, because however much we think we know where we are going, the unexpected frequently sends us off in a completely different direction. This has been particularly evident in my own life where an experience of medicine in South America landed me in gaol and then thrust me into the human rights struggle. Like Moses, my next Bible character, I couldn't have been more unsuitable for political work and yet my very naivety and ignorance gave my testimony a credibility it would have lacked had I been a political activist who 'got what was coming to her'.

Moses, if you remember, was a murderer: he found an Egyptian beating up an Israelite slave and, looking swiftly to left and to right to make sure no one was watching, did him in and buried him in the sand. The next day, however, Moses realised he had been spotted and departed speedily for the Sinai desert before the law could catch up with him. The omnipresent, inescapable God pursued him and called him by name one day as he was watching his father-in-law's goats. 'Moses!' said God, 'I have heard the cry of my people Israel and I am sending you to rescue them.' Moses, not surprisingly, was appalled and argued with God that he had a stammer and so would be useless at public speaking, not to mention his fear of flying, migraines or whatever it was that ailed him. Yahweh, however, would have none of it and sent him packing.

God makes no promise to those he sends that all will be well. Indeed no: the stories of malaria and martyrdom make that abundantly clear. The only promise he makes is the one he made to Abraham: 'I will be with you.' It seems to me vital that we take this on board. God, I believe, does not favour Christians any more than anyone else and he clearly does not exempt them from disease or disaster. *But*, if we call out his name, and if we listen, we will find that he is with us everywhere.

My third biblical call story is from chapter 6 of the prophet Isaiah and is the source of my theory about a wheelchair God. Isaiah is saying his prayers one day when he has an extremely scary vision of the Divine. In the midst of this experience, Isaiah hears God call, 'Whom shall I send?' This I see as the call made on behalf of all God's *anawim* – his broken people – whether they be refugees, famine victims, cancer patients or the mentally ill. God does not – cannot – feed the hungry, liberate the prisoner or bind up the hearts that are broken. Why? That is part of the Mystery and that is why I speak of a wheelchair God who cannot go himself, so he sends us, whoever will answer his call.

Isaiah, like Moses, like us, protested his unsuitability as a messenger: 'I am a man of unclean lips,' he said, 'and I come from a people of unclean lips.' God is not interested in our excuses, and, realising this, Isaiah finally says, 'Lord, if I'm any use to you, send me!'

Here we have my theology of call in a nutshell: God calls the unsuitable, by name, into the unknown, for a specific mission, which will be revealed when they arrive, wherever it is they are going. In exchange for their willingness to do his work, God makes a covenant with each person, just as he did with Noah after the flood. The covenant is that God will be with us, in sickness and in health, that we shall be his people and he will be our God. In Noah's case, God set a rainbow in the sky as a sign of this covenant: which is why, of course, I talk about the 'Theology of Rainbows'.

As time went by, after the retreat, I became more settled and content. I took on extra voluntary work at a shanty-town clinic and worked occasionally with Chris and his young Chilean 'disciples'. Three of these, young men in their early twenties, came to live in the upstairs of my house prior to entering the Jesuit novitiate. It was Chris's idea that they should experience looking after themselves, without the pampering of maids and mother, so that they might have some chance of surviving the rather 'basic' conditions of the novitiate. I was delighted to have their company, though on Chris's instructions they kept themselves to themselves. It was while the boys were living with me that I took the steps which were to lead me a little closer to conflict with the law.

Once every six days I worked the night at the Posta. The six teams normally worked a two-and-a-half-hour shift, mine being from around eleven until one-thirty in the afternoon. On the day after a team worked the night, their shift was covered by the *Volante* or 'Flying' shift which did a different time each day. On that particular night I was woken at 2 a.m. to see a patient. I came downstairs to hear a boy's voice crying, '*Maté un hombre*' – 'I killed a man, I killed a man.' The orderly led me from the distressed young soldier to the next room where, naked on the couch, lay the body of a boy around seventeen years old, rent apart by seven machine-gun bullets.

This was the closest that I had come to the horror of civil war and I felt both sick and enraged at the wanton destruction of a young life. Driven mad by impotence, I decided that the only thing I could do was record the boy's injuries in the cause of justice and somehow or other get word to his mother so that at least this man should not join the ranks of the disappeared.

The following day I made contact with the parish priest of the *poblacion* where the boy lived and, by pure serendipity, made the acquaintance of a man who was extremely active in human rights affairs in Chile. Father Fernando Salas was a Jesuit, a man in his thirties of upper-middle-class background who, along with the rest of his circle, had made a decision for a radical solidarity with the poor and oppressed. Much taken with him as a man and a priest, I invited him to take lunch with me one day in my house in the Calle Francisco Bilbao.

Some weeks later, Fernando came for his lunch date and, in a moment of bravura, I told him that I had returned to Chile because I knew that one day I'd be asked to treat a man with a bullet in his leg. Little did I know that, before many weeks had passed, Fernando himself would make that request of me.

During the retreat in Malloco I had seen my life as a blank cheque handed over willingly to God. Innocent that I was, I had no idea how soon and for how much that cheque would be drawn.

NOTES
1. See Karen Armstrong, *The Spiral Staircase* (HarperCollins, 2004).
2. Genesis 12.

14

⁓⊙⁓⊙⁓

ARREST AND TORTURE: OCTOBER 1974

B y now it was October 1974 and I was happily settled at work and in contact with many of the Santiago community of American missionaries. I was a frequent visitor at the Columban house and Bill Halliden, the superior of the community, was especially kind to me. My closest friends, however, were Ita, Carla and Rebecca, the Maryknoll sisters, as well as Jane, Connie and Liz. These women lived enormously dedicated lives under quite difficult circumstances and I often felt like an impostor in their company. How ironic it was, then, that it was I who fell foul of the law and ended up in detention.

One morning, quite early, I had a phone call from Fernando Salas asking me if he could visit, so I happily invited him to breakfast, looking forward to good conversation over toast and coffee. When he arrived, however, Fernando explained what he wanted of me: a number of left-wing freedom fighters had taken refuge in church property overnight and one of them had a bullet in his leg. How would I feel about attending to him medically? I was both scared and excited: here at last was the opportunity to prove my commitment to my friends, and surely, if I were caught, I would simply be deported. After all, no one would harm the daughter of a British Air Vice-Marshal. Anyway, there was no way I could refuse Fernando, so I said of course I would see the man.

When we got to the house of the two sisters of Notre Dame, where the fugitives were being sheltered, I found a man, Nelson Gutierrez, the second in command of the MIR (the Movement of the Revolutionary Left) and two women, Mariella Bachman and Mary Ann Beausire, whose brother William had been abducted by the DINA while on a business trip between Santiago and Buenos Aires. Mary Ann was the partner of Andres Pascal Allende, head of the MIR. The Beausires had English roots and William was one of a small number of English people who had suffered at the hands of the security forces.

The group had been surprised by the DINA in their hideout in Malloco; one man was shot dead, Nelson was wounded in the leg and the others escaped. Mariella, as she ran for her life, handed her baby to an unknown woman and was now distraught because she had no idea where the baby was. Mary Ann, however, was quite charming and came with me while I boiled my instruments on the kitchen stove.

Nelson I found to be a rather surly young man, huddled under the covers of his bed. He had sustained two bullet wounds in the calf and there was no way I could remove the bullets under these conditions. I suggested he should go into asylum so that he could get professional treatment, but he was adamant that he must stay where he was. All I could do was drain an abcess under local anaesthesia, dress the wounds and prescribe some antibiotics.

Next day, Nelson's condition was worse, despite the antibiotics. The man himself was feverish and I feared he would become delirious, so I explained to him that by refusing to go into asylum he could be putting his friends at risk. My medical authoritarian stance seemed to have worked, for Nelson eventually agreed to go into asylum in the *Nunciatura,* the house of the Papal Nuncio who had diplomatic status. I was greatly relieved when I heard this for I knew there was a limit to what I could do for him without hospital facilities. My relief, however, was to be short lived, for, a day or so later, I was summoned to meet with one of the bishops of Santiago.

All of this was distinctly cloak and dagger and appealed to my theatrical instincts. I met the bishop in a convent in Providencia, the up-market residential area of Santiago, and he asked me if I was prepared to attempt to remove the bullet from Nelson's leg. Now, I had been taught from my medical school days that it is serious folly to attempt to remove a 'foreign body' without X-ray control. I explained this to his Lordship but was told that there was absolutely no possibility of Nelson going to hospital because he would most certainly be arrested, tortured and killed. I thought about it and said that I would attempt it the following day but could not promise success. The next morning, therefore, I 'borrowed' an Esmark bandage from the Posta and prepared myself to do surgery. An Esmark bandage is a long strip of rubber which is wrapped around the limb in order to exsanguinate it: drive the blood back to the centre of the body. Only then would I have a chance of finding the foreign body for which I was searching.

I discussed the venture with Fernando and his fellow Jesuit, Father Patricio Cariola, and it was decided that I should go to the Nunciatura disguised as a nun and that I should call myself the Madre Isabella. The name was the somewhat humorous choice of the two men because Isabella is Spanish for Elizabeth, the Queen of England. That afternoon, therefore, I put on a skirt and went semi-demurely to call upon the Papal Nuncio. I was greeted by Monsignor Sergio Vallech, the Santiago 'Vicar for Religious', who walked me round the embassy grounds asking me what I was doing in Chile in general and mixed up in this business in particular.

When he had satisfied himself of my credentials, the Monsignor informed me that my services would not be needed, and bid me goodbye. I was both thankful and a little put out, having been thwarted in my heroic act of mercy, and returned home to shed the identity of the Madre Isabella and reclaim my own as the *gringa* doctor with the three chows. I thought no more about Nelson and his friends and happily picked up the threads of my life.

Down the road, at the house of the Columban Fathers, there was a visitor in the form of Sister Connie Kelly of the New York Sisters of Charity. Connie had been working too hard in the *poblacion* where she lived and was in need of rest and recuperation. She went initially to the Maryknoll house in the Calle Los Leones but continued to be high as a kite, talking for hours to anyone who came to see her. It was decided, therefore, that she should spend a week in the Columbans' house as only Bill Halliden and the bursar lived there full time. I was asked to keep a friendly medical eye on her so I visited a couple of times a day.

On a Saturday evening, it was 1 November, I was sitting chatting with Connie in her bedroom while Bill Halliden was in his office, preparing his sermon for the following day. Suddenly, there was a shot, and a scream from Enriquetta, the Columbans' maid, and both Bill and I rushed to the head of the stairs to see what was happening. To our horror, we came upon the prone figure of Enriquetta lying on the floor with a bullet hole in her back. We rushed to her side and were suddenly assailed by a hail of gunfire from outside the house. Between us, we tried to pull Enriquetta into the shelter of the corridor, then fled for our lives and crouched under the kitchen table.

Bill was desperate to give Enriquetta the last rites and, had I not stopped him, would have gone out to his car for the holy oils. I looked frantically around the kitchen and my eyes fixed upon a large pot of Nivea hand cream and I wondered briefly whether this would serve his purpose. I decided, regretfully, that Nivea was probably not mentioned in canon law and suggested cooking oil instead. It's hard to explain how I felt to be in the midst of this drama, which was for all the world like a bad B movie. I was scared, and my mind raced, trying to think who it might be that was attacking this quiet, religious house.

After a while the shooting ceased and a number of men entered the room. They asked my name and, when I told them, one man said to another, '*Esta ella estamos buscando!*' 'She's the one we're looking for.' It still didn't occur to me that this was the dreaded security police, the DINA or Directorate of National Intelligence. In my innocence I wondered if they were the MIR come to carry me off to treat some other wounded fugitive. Whoever they were, I wanted nothing to do with them and crept upstairs and locked myself in the bathroom. As soon as they realised I was missing, however, there was much shouting and rushing about, then a loud knocking on the bathroom door with threats that they would shoot me if I didn't come out.

Reluctantly, I emerged and was led downstairs and out of the house, past a terrified Mercedes who was sitting on the doorstep. It turned out that the DINA had gone first to my house and arrested two of the three would-be seminarians before persuading Mercedes to tell them where I was. This was the beginning of a nightmare experience in captivity which was to end two months later with my expulsion from Chile as an unwanted person and a political activist. The daft thing was, I was never politically active: all I had done was accede to a priest's request to treat a wounded man.

As they pushed me into a waiting car, one of the men gave me a slap across the face before tying a blindfold around my eyes. I was outraged at this gratuitous violence, for what had I ever done to hurt them? Then we set off, at high speed, through the darkened city towards the mountains. After about twenty minutes, or perhaps more, we slowed down and I heard the clang of iron gates: the gates, I was soon to learn, of the Villa Grimaldi, an old farm which had been taken over by the DINA as an interrogation centre.

Within minutes of my arrival I was hustled into a small room containing several men and a metal bunk bed without a mattress. Without preamble I was ordered to remove my clothes and when I demurred the man grabbed at my shirt, tearing it a little. I protested that I was British and the daughter of a high-ranking military officer but they simply laughed and said that their image abroad was of no importance to them. I was then forced down on to the bed and spread-eagled, naked on the bare springs, secured by ties around wrists and ankles and a band over my belly. I was blindfolded and then the electric shocks began – delivered through electrodes which they moved over my body. After they had given me a taste of the pain, they demanded that I tell them who had asked me to treat Gutierrez.

Anxious to defend Fernando and Patricio, I said it was a man I had met at a party. They continued: 'Where did the man live?' At this stage of the interrogation there was enough time between the shocks for me to invent my story, so I said the man lived in a big white house with black wrought-iron gates in a street called Bishop something or other. The men talked excitedly among themselves, clearly believing that they had extracted valuable information from me. Then, mercifully, the shocks stopped and they told me to get dressed. Stiffly and painfully I put on my clothes, and this time I was taken to a van and told to get into the front seat. Then the driver and another man got in and we drove off at high speed to the south of the city. Thankful as I was to be free of the pain, I realised that they would be furious with me when they discovered that I had been lying. Then, to my horror, they stopped in front of a large white house with black gates and I saw the street sign: it was Obispo Subercaseaux, Bishop Subercaseaux. The men demanded to know if this was the house and I said I thought it was. Jubilant, they sent for back-up, and took me with them as they waited in the street. As we stood there, two men passed by and, desperate, I shouted to them, 'Help! I'm a prisoner of the DINA.' I grabbed hold of the man's jacket but he pulled free and hurried down the street with his friend without a backward glance: sensible Chileans did not play the hero with the DINA. My captors were furious and one man said coldly, 'It would be much easier if we killed you now.'

When back-up arrived the men entered the house dragging me with them. At first I was hopeful that the owners would be cultured people who would understand English and take pity on me but, to my horror, there was only an elderly couple, caretakers of an empty house in which all the furniture was draped in sheets. The old man and his wife were terrified as the men questioned them and, fearing for their safety, I told my captors that I had lied to them, that this was not the house. Once they believed me, I was taken back to the van and returned to the Villa Grimaldi.

Back on the 'parrilla', the barbecue as they called it, my treatment was much harsher than before. This time I was gagged and they put an electrode in my vagina so that the shocks affected my whole body and were much more severe. They resumed their interrogation, telling me to raise a finger when I was ready to answer. The pain was a nightmare and they delivered the shocks with such rapidity that I was quite unable to fabricate another story. In a cruel twist, they ignored my signals so that each time I tried to speak they kept on with the shocks. Eventually, I told them that I had been asked to treat Gutierrez by a priest and that he had been sheltered in a convent of American nuns. Once again, they took me out to identify the house where the nuns lived but they kept me in the car while they went in to search it. The men, however, were more perplexed then ever as the owners of the convent were away and it was being looked after by other nuns from a different congregation! I was returned once more to the Grimaldi and the *parilla* and, around seven in the morning, I told them the names of the priests involved, calculating that I had given them eight hours in which to go into hiding. I was sad but not ashamed that I had not held out longer; I did what I could and that was that.

When the interrogation was over I was taken to a room where I met three young women, university students who had also been interrogated. Never have women seemed more like angels: they were so kind and gentle with me, helping me onto a bunk. I was thirsty but they told me I must drink nothing for twenty-four hours because of the electricity. I was so frightened and lay on the bunk wondering what would happen next.

I spent three days at the Grimaldi: plenty of time to get to know my companions. The youngest was Flavia, who was only seventeen; the others were in their twenties. After twenty-four hours we were joined by another girl, Leilia, also a youngster, who was full of rebellious spirit despite having been rendered deaf in one ear by 'the telephones' (simultaneous blows to the ears). There were many different methods of torture: some people were half drowned when their heads were submerged in a bucket of faecally contaminated water, others were suspended from poles, attacked by dogs and, of course, most of the women had been raped.

There were men, too, in the Grimaldi. We counted fifty of them as they walked in single file, blindfold, to the lavatory, each with a hand on the shoulder of the man in front. One morning we sang to the men as they passed by our window: the *Cancion a La Alegria*, Beethoven's *Hymn to Joy*. Another day we heard a man being interrogated in the room next door and then one of the guards brought in a blood-stained shirt and asked one of the girls to wash it.

I was acutely aware of God during those three days: but it was a powerless God, suffering with me, not a rescuer. I longed to leave my mark upon this hateful place and as I lay on my lower bunk I made a cross on the supports of the bunk above my head, pulling black wool from the blanket and binding it on to the crossed metal bands.

By the third day I felt quite a bit better and I was told to leave the room. One of the terrifying things about the Grimaldi was that they deliberately, I'm sure, never told us where they were taking us or what was to happen next. Each time, therefore, I was taken away from the girls I was completely terrified. On the last day I was blindfolded with Scotch tape so that I could see absolutely nothing. They put a pair of dark glasses on my face and told me to stand still. Then I heard the engine of a large vehicle rev up and come towards me; I thought wildly, 'O my God, they're going to run me over!' As the terror rose in my throat the engine slowed down and stopped and I was ordered to get into the vehicle. Like all the men and women driven away from the Grimaldi into the unknown, I did not know if I was being taken to some lonely hillside to be shot or to somewhere to be released.

I was, in fact, being transferred to another detention centre, Cuatro Alamos, the Four Poplars, which was a place of solitary confinement on the other side of the city where prisoners were kept until the information they had divulged under torture was verified. On arrival, I was taken to my 'cell': a narrow room with two bunks and a barred window looking out onto the foothills of the Andes. This, though I did not know it then, was to be my home for the next three weeks.

15

SOLITARY CONFINEMENT

Solitary confinement was not in itself terrifying but the fear seized me every time I heard the key turn in the lock and subsided when the door was closed again. There were, however, many hardships and the humiliation of having to pee into a small tin can because I had no free access to a lavatory. The vaginal electrodes had left me with a severe urethritis, so that I felt the need to urinate almost continually.

The other hardship was the poor quality of the food: we were given dry bread and tea for breakfast, soup and bread for lunch and some kind of pasta for supper. The poorer prisoners no doubt took this in their stride but I found the bread stuck in my throat and I could not continue eating for fear that I would vomit. I lost a stone during my time in prison.

I saw nothing of the other prisoners though I heard them and there was some communication between the cells by banging the wall or the window bars. We were allowed no exercise, minimal washing facilities and no change of clothing. My jeans, soaked with Enriquetta's blood and my own, were filthy and my underclothes simply disintegrated.

Within a few days I had a visit from Derek Fernyhough, the British Consul, but we were supervised by the camp commander who insisted that we speak in Spanish. Afraid of retribution, I said that I was fine and that I had been well treated, but there was a brief moment when the governor was distracted and I tried to get across to Derek that I had been tortured by saying 'Mains, Derek, mains', hoping that he would understand what I meant as I dare not say 'electricity' as it is too close to the Spanish word *electricidad*. Derek told me that my arrest was big news in the UK and that the Foreign Office was negotiating actively with the Chilean government for my release.

I spent three weeks in solitary confinement in Cuatro Alamos, a time marked by great fear and a massive spiritual struggle to accept what was happening to me with grace and dignity. My first instinct was to scream at God to be let out. 'Lord! Help! Get me out of here!' was my unspoken cry as I metaphorically beat my hands against the bars of my prison. Little by little, however, it occurred to me that there was a better way and I struggled to pray that God's will be done. The prayer learned in childhood, 'Grant that I may love you always – then do with me what you will', became my own as I fought to make sense of what was happening to me. This act of abandonment to the will of God was for me an enormously powerful religious experience of which the retreat in Malloco seems to have been a prelude. During that retreat I had drawn a picture of a cheque which read 'Payable to God, one life' and signed 'Sheila Cassidy'. Now in this bleak prison it seemed that God had taken me at my word. There were times when I felt strong enough to hand the cheque over – and others when I snatched it back and ripped it into a dozen pieces.

There was a particular night when the struggle reached its climax: I had been taken before the Prosecutor Fiscal, the military prosecutor, and had learned that I was to be charged with killing Enriquetta, the Columban Fathers' maid. The DINA, it seemed, were convinced that I had had an accomplice and that Enriquetta had been killed in the crossfire, a story which exonerated them of the murder of an innocent mother of two. When I asked the Fiscal what was to happen to me, he said that I would be tried and, if found guilty, I would be sentenced, possibly to life imprisonment. I can't remember if he said that I might be sentenced to death but I know I thought that that was a possibility.

I lay awake all night thinking of what he had said and argued with the God to whom I had so foolishly handed over my life.

'I thought you wanted me to be a nun,' I said.

I suspect God grinned and said, 'I thought you made me a gift of yourself.'

'Yes,' I said, 'but . . . '

'Well?'

On it went, all night, until wearily, in the early hours, I handed over my crumpled, tear-stained cheque: to God, one life.

The drama which I have recounted is a story of an act of abandonment to the will of God, and it is no coincidence that I had been given a copy of Father Edward Farrell's *Disciples and Other Strangers* (Denville NJ:

Dimension Books, 1974), which contained an anonymous poem about abandonment. I do not have it to hand as I write but I remember the following lines:

> Abandonment is not the act of a child . . .
> It is a letting go of the strings by which we manipulate our lives . . .
> It is the climactic moment of any man's life.

Looking back over the past thirty years, I believe that this was indeed for me a climactic moment, for however I may have strayed from the straight and narrow, since then, I have been possessed of a kind of peace about the future. I believe at a very deep level that God has his/her world in hand and that, as Julian of Norwich said so long ago, 'All things shall be well; all things shall be well and all manner of things shall be well.'

It is important to say that this trust in God is not to be equated with a naive belief that God will protect me from harm. Ten years of depression during my years at the hospice and bilateral breast cancer in 2002 has taught me that I am as vulnerable as the next woman. During these times of suffering and difficulty I have, I think, always known that God was there, with me, sharing my experience. This was not necessarily an immediate comfort: it did not take away the despair of insomnia, nor the sadness of losing my breasts, but it gave me strength to endure.

On the second day that I went before the Fiscal I explained to him that I was terrified in the hands of the DINA: afraid that I would be returned to the Grimaldi for further interrogation. He arranged, therefore, for me to be transferred to the Casa de Correction for women: the women's common gaol where, he said, I would be under his jurisdiction and, therefore, safe. That afternoon, I was taken to the women's prison where, to my astonishment, I was welcomed by a group of nuns! The women's prison, it emerged, was run by the Good Shepherd nuns who were founded to care for 'fallen women'.

The sisters welcomed me warmly and I was led down various corridors until we arrived at a small office where I was introduced to two young women prisoners and, amazingly, a box of baby ducklings! The two young women had belonged to an extra-radical political party and had been in detention since the coup. They were quite charming and I spent an hour or so with them until I was told I must be locked up for the night. The nun led me through the prison, past a number of 'ordinary' prisoners, until we arrived at a small cell whose only window was onto the main dormitory in which it was situated. As the key turned in the lock

I was once more lonely and afraid and conscious that I had less space now than I had had at Cuatro Alamos.

The following day I was driven once more to the basement court where the Fiscal was now interviewing Fernando and Patricio, the two Jesuits who had first asked me to treat Gutierrez. To my horror they were in leg irons, but these were soon removed and Fernando and I managed to talk to each other by walking across the room in opposite directions and talking softly each time we passed.

Towards the end of the day, the Fiscal called me in and said that the charges against me were to be dropped and that I was free to go. I was astonished and jubilant but Fernando and Patricio were deeply worried and saw this as an opportunity for the DINA to seize me and make me disappear. In fact, I was never released, for my captors said I had to go back to the prison to be 'signed out'. When we were back at the prison they told me that the office was shut and that, it being Friday, I would have to remain in detention until Monday. I had been joined at the prison by Derek Fernyhough, the British Consul and a human rights lawyer who spent over an hour on the telephone trying fruitlessly to secure my release.

When the Fiscal said I could go home I somehow dropped my guard, so when told that I must wait over the weekend I broke down and wept. I had held myself together for so long but now I had had enough and I made quite a scene. Eventually, the lawyer told me I must pull myself together or the police would think I had something to hide and might decide to interrogate me again. Crushed beyond words, I regained my cool and watched with grave foreboding as Derek and the lawyer left.

The following day, the DINA came for me again and I was taken back to my cell at Cuatro Alamos where I spent a further ten days in detention. The prison must have been filling up, for, after a week, I was joined, first by Lelia whom I had met at the Grimaldi and then by an older woman, Adriana, who had also been tortured. Lelia and I spoke for hours and developed a strong bond despite the twenty years' age gap between us. She knew all about the political detention system and told me that next door to the solitary confinement block there was the camp of Tres Alamos, the Three Poplars, where over six hundred political prisoners were held. Once prisoners were transferred there the military admitted that they were being held, whereas those of us in solitary were still 'disappeared' and, therefore, very much more at risk. I later learned that some prisoners who were seen at the Grimaldi and again in Cuatro Alamos did not make it to the more open prison and were never seen again. Over two thousand men and women disappeared in the wake of the coup and were eventually presumed dead.

One such woman was the mother of one of the younger prisoners who, on her way to visit her daughter at Tres Alamos, found a left-wing flier in the street. Thinking it would interest her daughter she popped it in her bag where it was discovered when her things were searched at visiting time. Despite her protests, she was taken to the Grimaldi to be interrogated because no one believed her story that she was an ordinary, rather right-wing housewife. She was seen by two other prisoners at the Grimaldi but never arrived at Tres Alamos and was not seen again.

I, however, was lucky because towards the end of November I was transferred to Tres Alamos.

16

─◦◦─◦◦─

TRES ALAMOS:
NOVEMBER 1975

I think it is true to say that my time in Tres Alamos detention camp was one of the richest experiences of my life. When the time came for me to leave Cuatro Alamos, the prison chief led me down a short corridor and opened a gate to reveal a sea of smiling faces. These were the young women, branded as Marxist terrorists and held in detention because they posed a threat to the security of the state. Never have I received such a welcome: arms were outstretched to embrace me, faces to kiss me, and I was offered delicacies such as fruit and yoghurt. It had never occurred to me that I had achieved fame in Chile: that I would go down in history as the *gringa* who had endured torture because she had treated a wounded man. The women thanked me again and again for what I had done for their people and one woman wrote me the most amazing poem: a eulogy in honour of my solidarity.

The gesture I remember most, however, was when Anita Maria, seeing me wrestling with my unkempt hair which kept falling over my eyes, quietly removed her own hair grip and handed it to me. That is generosity indeed: giving away what one needs oneself rather than out of one's excess. I learned so much about giving and sharing from these young women who lived an Acts of the Apostles style of life in common. At the end of every visiting session all food and gifts were pooled. They made yoghurt from powdered milk donated by the Red Cross and gave that to the weakest as there was not sufficient for all.

The work too was shared, food prepared, floors swept and lavatories cleaned. In addition to the housework there were a number of craft projects: leather work, embroidery and carving in bone. This last they had developed to an art form: little doves of peace or crosses were cut with a hacksaw out of beef bones, filed and sanded smooth and then polished with toothpaste. I made two crosses for my friends Ita and Carla and, to my amazement, one of the men made one for me. Each day two girls were taken to the men's side of the camp to fetch the lunchtime soup and this brief encounter was taken advantage of to exchange notes and small gifts. One day the girls brought me back two miniature brass chalices, turned on a lathe. They were exquisitely beautiful and I treasure them to this day.

Another art form was the making of beads from dry bread. I have two sets of these: dark, plain beads made by Sara while she was in solitary and brightly coloured painted ones made in Tres Alamos itself. I enjoyed myself greatly trying out the different crafts, and people made things for me. I still have a pair of sandals with soles made out of car tyres, a leather belt and a cover for the psalm book given me by one of the nuns.

It was much harder to pray in Tres Alamos than when I had been in solitary because I had virtually no time to myself. I shared a six-foot-square room with five other women; though, at one time when the camp was overcrowded, someone had to sleep on the floor as well. The volunteer for this uncomfortable position was medical student Christina Zamorra whose partner was also detained in a prison many miles out of Santiago. Christina later came to the UK and qualified as a doctor. Beatriz Miranda, a delightful high-spirited young woman, slept in the bunk above me and I used to poke her between the slats which formed the bed to wake her in the morning. Beatriz also came to the UK and married an English doctor. They have two little girls and are well settled in the UK. Beatriz worked as a lab technician and has recently qualified as a counsellor.

Everyone was so friendly and concerned for my well-being that any time I tried to escape from company they thought I was unhappy and came to cheer me up. I would protest that I liked to be alone but they found that morbid and engaged me in conversation.

There were two women who had been in the camp much longer than the others: Luz de las Nieves Ayres and an older woman, a journalist called Gladys Diaz. Luz had been in Tres Alamos for over two years and believed she would never be let out because of the testimony she could give of particularly bestial torture involving rats and dogs. Her grandfather was Scots and she was applying for asylum in the UK, although she

was eventually released to East Germany. Gladys Diaz was an exceptionally strong woman who was said to have held out longer under torture
than anyone else. She was also a senior member of the MIR and was held
in awe by many of the younger prisoners.

Twice a week we were allowed visitors and were taken through the
camp to an area of grass where everyone sat and talked urgently to their
friends and relatives. I was delighted to have lots of visitors: Ita and Carla,
Jane and Liz and several of the Columban priests. I remember particularly Peter Murphy, a warm-hearted Australian, with whom I had worked
to try and improve the diet in the children's soup kitchens. I was to meet
up with him in Brisbane many years later. I had told some of the nuns
that I missed being able to go to Mass and after that someone always
brought me a consecrated host. Sometimes more than one person
brought it and I was able to keep the hosts and receive communion each
morning when I woke. I kept the hosts in my toiletry bag and would
unzip it with infinite care lest I wake one of my room-mates.

There was no religious input to the camp and a small group of us
decided to ask the camp commander if a priest could celebrate Mass for
us. At first it seemed there was no possibility and some of the women
asked me to hold a service for them, which I did. At Christmas, however,
we were allowed a priest to celebrate Mass and I have fond memories of
Maria Bernales, a woman from the country and author of my poem,
taking her newborn baby Xaviera up for a blessing. Twenty years later I
was lecturing in Toronto only to find that Xaviera was one of the young
women performing a dance that night!

As Christmas approached, the possibility of my release was increasingly mentioned on the radio and my hopes were raised. A few days
before, Reggie Seconde, the British Ambassador to Chile, came to visit me
bearing a tinned Christmas cake and a jar of butterscotch sweets from
Harrods. I fell upon the sweets and looked forward to sharing them and
the cake with my special friends, especially Beatriz. I pictured her tasting
the cake and exclaiming that she had never tasted anything so delicious.
When I offered them, however, Beatriz would have none of it and said I
should hand everything in to the food pool. I was appalled: how far
would one jar of sweets go around eighty women, let alone a small cake?
I pressed the sweets upon her and, reluctantly, she took one, only to
bitterly regret it later and reproach me for seducing her away from her
principles. We both ended up in tears and, with extreme ill grace, I
handed both the sweets and the cake into the pool.

The following day was Christmas Eve and there were furious preparations for the party to be held that night. The fate of my poor Christmas cake, the only Harrods cake I'd ever had, made my hair stand on end for they mixed it with quantities of caramelised condensed milk to make a pudding to feed all eighty of us: a true miracle of the loaves and fishes. That evening everyone put on their best clothes and we gathered to drink fruit punch and eat *empanados*, the traditional Chilean pies which appear whenever there is a celebration. Alas, there were no pisco sour cocktails, the unique mixture of concentrated grape liquor and lemon juice!

After we had eaten, there occurred the most moving concert that I have ever experienced: the women sang for their menfolk, imprisoned the other side of the wall. Climbing up on benches and tables so that their voices would carry further, they sang as if their lungs would burst until, in the distance, we heard the faint sound of men's voices singing in reply. In my heart, I still hear the echo of their favourite song, 'Animo! Negro Jose!' – 'Take heart, Joe, my love'.

I had wanted so badly to be home for Christmas but I am glad now that I spent that time with my friends. They were an amazing group of young women, mostly students in their early twenties who had become aware of the injustice in their country while doing placements with the poor. There were medical students like Cristina, the midwife Susanna Veraguas, social workers, psychologists and more. Never before or since have I been privileged to spend time with such idealistic and courageous young women. There was a generosity of spirit and a compassion in these women which, alas, I did not find in the nuns when, eventually, I entered the convent. These women may have been ideologically Marxist but their behaviour was truly Christian.

Christmas week dragged by without news but, the day before New Year's Eve, there was word on the radio that I was due to be expelled from the country the following day. High on anticipation, I packed my few possessions and the women prepared messages for me to take to England, concealed about my person. The first was a list of all the women who had applied for British visas, which they copied onto the inside of the waist-band of my jeans. (Within two weeks I was able to read from this list in the office of the Foreign Secretary while a secretary copied it down onto his notepad.) The second was the poem written for me by Maria Bernales, which they wrote on the fabric hidden by the turn-ups of my jeans. The third message was the most important and caused me considerable anxiety as it was a highly confidential message to be delivered to someone on the plane.

Although the women put on such a brave face, they were in fact very frightened that the authorities were to simulate a mass escape which they would use as the opportunity to kill a large number of the women. 'Shot while trying to escape' is a classic excuse for getting rid of tiresome prisoners. Some of the women had heard strange noises in the night and there was a rumour that the authorities were digging a tunnel under the camp as evidence of the break-out. As things turned out, I was unable to deliver the message because the person to whom it was addressed was not on the plane and I felt enormously guilty when I arrived in Devon with the vital message written on green silk in the waistband of my jeans.

The following day, the Camp Commander arrived and peremptorily ordered the women to go to the place where we normally received our visitors. I was about to follow them when he called me and told me that I was leaving and I had three minutes to pack. Still unable to believe that I might soon be free, I packed my belongings and told the guard I was ready. Then to my horror I was led into a building and taken downstairs into a basement room. I was terrified and thought that they were going to shoot me now and tell all my friends that I had returned to England. I need not have worried, however, for they had brought me here to sign a form saying that I had been well treated and that I had not been submitted to torture or any inhuman treatment during my stay in Tres and Cuatro Alamos. Then they carefully searched my bags and confiscated some sketches which I had made of my fellow prisoners and of the camp itself. At last, they were finished and we returned upstairs where I was handed over to a strange man in a suit who said he would be accompanying me to the airport.

Once more I was deeply afraid, for I had thought that the Consul would come with me. The stranger explained that he was from the CIME, the International Committee for Refugees, but I had never heard of it and I didn't believe him. Once again I thought that I was to be driven to some barren spot and shot in cold blood.

If my fears seem neurotic, it is as well to remember the two thousand disappeared Chileans as well as a small number of foreigners, all of whom were murdered in cold blood. One of these was a Catholic priest, Father Michael Woodward, who was tortured and killed aboard the training ship *Esmeralda* in the harbour of Valparaiso during the early days of the coup. Michael's story is recorded by Father Edward Creuzet in his book *Death on the Esmeralda*. The other well-known case is that of the young American who is the subject of the well-known film *Missing*. Once again I realise how lucky I was to escape with my life and as few scars as I had.

Eventually, we arrived at Santiago's airport of Pudahuel and I was led onto the tarmac to meet the Consul and the Ambassador who had come to see me off. It is worth recording here that, at his last meeting with me at Tres Alamos, Mr Seconde had strongly advised me that, when I returned to England, I should keep my mouth shut and not talk to the press. His reasoning was that it would be much better for me to recuperate quietly in the bosom of my family. I initially accepted his advice but when I told my fellow prisoners about this they were appalled.

I was taken for an interview with Gladys Diaz who let me know in no uncertain terms that they were counting on me to broadcast their story to the entire world. I was their only hope of getting the international publicity which would, they hoped, protect them and lead eventually to their getting visas to leave the country. I took in what she said, and promised that I would do everything in my power. Gladys herself was eventually deported to the GDR, along with 'Light of the Snows', Luz de las Nieves Ayres.

At last, I was led by the man from the CIME towards the aeroplane. As I walked I heard my name called and, there on the spectators' balcony, were my friends the missionaries who had come to bid me farewell. I have a photograph of myself waving ecstatically to them, accompanied by a tight-lipped, serious man who was clearly desperate to get me to the safety of the aircraft. Finally, I was on board and settled into a window seat, with my Chilean poncho and a shirt embroidered for me by the women.

Then, at last, we took off and I gazed with tears in my eyes as Chile and my friends disappeared from view. It was 30 December 1975 and I was scheduled to arrive at London's Heathrow on New Year Eve.

17

RETURN TO ENGLAND: 1976

It is difficult to articulate my feelings as the plane took off and I looked down for what I thought was to be the last time at Chile. I felt overwhelmed by a mixture of joy and sadness and could not quite take in the fact that I was free at last.

Even the word *free* seems wrong for I realised now that no one who experiences what I underwent in Chile can ever be the same again. It is not just the torture, or the overwhelming fear, that branded me, but the inescapable fact of having been caught up in history, marked out for some curious mission. It is as though what happened to me was somehow planned, all the ingredients pre-selected to give me a particular role in the United Kingdom on behalf of the Chilean prisoners. As I said earlier, if the DINA authorities had realised how articulate I was, they would never have let me go.

They could have said I had been run over, killed in a confrontation with the police – whatever. There would have been outrage, of course, but there would have been many in Chile and in the UK who would have said that I was a poor misguided woman who got herself involved in politics. It would have hit all the newspapers for a couple of days, and then that would have been that. As things turned out, however, they saw me as a bedraggled figure, in my jeans and Peruvian sweater, and judged me to be a Marxist agitator who no one would believe.

But, from the very beginning, there were many who did believe my story, starting with Peter Birkett from the *Daily Mail* who flew with me from Santiago and Frank Taylor from the *Guardian* who joined us in Buenos Aires. The chief steward moved me up into first class to protect me from the press, but eventually I felt ready to talk and told them my story. This was the first real intimation I had of the impact that my story was to have in the UK and the beginning of my understanding of how I could use my own story on behalf of those I had left behind in prison. I talked to Peter and Frank all the way from Buenos Aires to Rio and they rushed off the plane to phone their 'copy' to their respective newspapers, only to be thwarted and told that they could not disembark and must return to Europe! I found their frustration very funny and we spent the rest of the flight sharing supper and drinking champagne to celebrate my freedom. Even as we laughed and drank, however, the memory of the women I'd left behind was with me. I longed to share my dinner with them and I was haunted by their fear and the danger they were in.

After Rio we flew to Madrid where, as in Buenos Aires and Rio, I was allowed off the plane but not into the airport lounge, as they were still afraid that the DINA might come after me. If that seems far-fetched, it is as well to remember that William Beausire was snatched somewhere on his flight to Buenos Aires and later seen in one of the Chilean secret houses by political prisoner Adriana Borquez, a remarkable social worker who lived south of Santiago in the city of Talca.

My arrival at Heathrow is a moment I shall never forget. I was asked to wait until the other passengers had disembarked and was just combing my hair when I was greeted by my brother Mike who had been allowed on the plane to see me, away from the glare of the cameras. I don't think I ever gave any thought to the anguish of my poor family who had no means of knowing whether or not I had become a terrorist, against all their conservative ideals. Mike and I faced the cameras together and were blinded by the battery of flashlights. We were led quickly to a VIP lounge and there, to my delight, I found a welcoming committee of friends and family. There was Father Michael Hollings, my number-one ecclesiastical hero from Oxford days, and Chilean friends Dr Alfredo Jadresic and a psychiatrist friend of Consuelo, Sonia Abovitch. Also there was my solicitor Neil from Leicester, determined to see that I did not commit myself to any newspaper deal without his approval. He assured me that I was free to walk away without giving the press an interview, but I knew that my obligations to my fellow prisoners demanded that I do that. I told him, therefore, that I wished to speak to all the press together and arrangements were made for me to go before the cameras, boasting proudly that I was not afraid of anyone who was not carrying a machine gun. This piece of bravado was typical of those early days back in the UK; I was high on the exhilaration of being free and on a powerful sense of mission to obtain the release of my fellow prisoners. I was also possessed of a kind of religious zeal, for the time in prison, especially in solitary, had been a very powerful spiritual experience.

On the day after my return, my brother's house in Devon, where I was staying, was besieged by reporters. My sister-in-law Pat, an ex-nurse, kept them at bay until after I had been to Mass, and then I met them. I had turned down all offers of exclusive stories the day before and given a general press conference. The *Sunday Mirror* still wanted an exclusive, so, thinking that 11 million readers would read my story, I signed a contract with them. For the next two weeks I had my own private reporter and photographer in attendance and felt like a film star. I walked by the sea with Ian Bradshaw doing the now familiar photographer's patter: 'Look left. Look this way. Chin up! Smile! Not so wide. Serious now. Smile. That's lovely', etc. etc. Meanwhile, David Duffy the reporter sat at the dining-room table tapping out my story on his portable typewriter. (No laptops in the 1970s!) The whole family joined in the drama and we have some wonderful photos of the children with which to remember those days.

When Duffy's articles were published on two consecutive Sundays I blushed at the headlines. 'Clockwork Orange House of Terror' was one of them; I forget the others. The response from the wider family was mixed: my cousin Julia remarked that she had put the paper on the floor but the dog wouldn't pee on it! Now, thirty years older, I am much more realistic about the gulf between Left and Right. One person's freedom fighter is another person's terrorist, and passionate witness on behalf of the oppressed can be seen by some as undignified exhibitionism. I remember my astonishment when, after a controversial TV programme when I was faced with a very right-wing Anglo-Chilean woman who said I was lying, the telephone lines to the BBC were blocked, 50 per cent in my favour and 50 per cent against. It was the same with the 'fan' mail, of which I received a fair amount. For some people I was a tortured heroine, for others a lying Marxist. The letter which said, 'I could tell by your lovely blue eyes that you were speaking the truth,' was balanced by the one which said, 'I could tell by looking at your eyes that you were lying!' At first, such letters used to hurt, but as time went by I learned to bin them. With hindsight, the most important thing for me personally about the *Mirror* reporters was that they fended off all other press invaders and I was protected and entertained for those crucial first two weeks.

When the *Mirror* reporters returned to London I embarked upon a one-woman crusade of human rights, lecturing passionately in an attempt to secure the freedom of Beatriz, Sara, Christina and all those whom I had left behind. Within a week I was speaking at the United Nations Assembly in Geneva and went from there to the House of Commons and to a number of universities. I appeared on various TV programmes and preached in cathedrals all over the UK. Looking back on those days, my memories are a kaleidoscope of fun and fear, exhilaration and exhaustion. There was no doubt that, like my father before me, I had a gift for public speaking and I used it ruthlessly in the cause of raising awareness of the plight of the Chilean political prisoners. In those early months I became widely known as 'the doctor who had been tortured in Chile', a title which I still bear nearly thirty years later. At the time I took it all in my stride, not seeking publicity but, if it came my way, ready to use it on behalf of the cause.

During the months to follow, my engagements were so varied that I found myself playing a number of different roles. In Geneva I was the guest of the British Ambassador and had to mind my manners, while on a tour of the Scandinavian countries I lectured to doctors and members of parliament, preached in the cathedral in Uppsala and spoke in Spanish at meetings of Chilean refugees and human rights activists. The latter engagements were by far the most fun. The halls (in Stockholm, Copenhagen and Oslo) were packed with students and refugees and my appearances were accompanied by a Chilean folk group which had happened to be out of Chile at the time of the coup and was now unable to return. We all raised the roof singing 'Venceremos!', the Chilean equivalent of 'We shall overcome', while the children ran backwards and forwards as children do.

During this trip my sister-in-law Pat and I were accompanied by a delightful Chilean called Daniel who had been in exile since the coup and who spoke good Swedish. At one stage of our travels we met an ardent Chilean Pentecostal metal worker who presented me with a wonderful wrought-iron crucifix. This was not a sentimental religious object by any means but a stark figure with fist raised to heaven crying for justice. I carried this object round Scandinavia, brandishing it like a battering ram as we ran for ferries and rushed from engagement to engagement. I remember too Daniel's patience when I realised I had left it behind on one of the ferries and he had to go back for it!

Pat's job on our tour was to support and protect me and there was a memorable day when she came to my rescue in Oslo. I had given a press conference that lasted two hours and went on way past my lunch hour. (I should explain that all Cassidys become extremely ratty if not fed regularly.) When told there was no time for lunch I gave a howl and flung my Bible against the wall, narrowly missing a kindly Lutheran minister! Pat sprang to my rescue: 'Now you've done it!' she said. 'You've broken her!' She explained tersely that I needed feeding, and after a few minutes a hamburger and a glass of milk were passed gingerly round the door! Once restored, we set out again and I was hustled protesting past enticing shops towards our next engagement with a Roman Catholic bishop. To my amazement, he looked kindly at me and asked, 'How are you?', at which I burst into tears!

After the Scandinavian trip came one to Paris. I have a clear memory of a kindly hostess who plied me with strong black coffee first thing in the morning when all I wanted was a very British cup of tea. Some time later came a trip to Finland where I gave evidence at a tribunal investigating the crimes of the military junta in Chile. My memory of this trip is of the static electricity of the hotel door handles which reminded me of the torture and being woken at three in the morning by Nelson Gutierrez who had phoned, not to say thank you but to ask who had betrayed me. I find it quite funny that all the pain and fear I endured was for the sake of a rather surly little man whom I wouldn't recognise if I met him in the street. But then charm and the finer points of etiquette are not part of the job description for Latin American revolutionaries.

Quite early on in that year of 1976 it was suggested that I write a short paperback on my experiences in Chile. I was asked to write an outline and when I had done that my agent sent a copy to the publishers of Collins books, as well as to Penguin. I was invited to meet Lady Collins in London and I can remember the pure exhilaration that I felt when I gave directions to the taxi driver as we set off for St James's Place. I leaned back in the taxi and watched London go by, pretending to myself that I was a writer on my way to my publisher. Lady Collins was a tiny, elderly woman who gave me tea in a bone china cup and was much concerned with serving milky tea in a bone china saucer to an elderly Pekinese. At first we made polite conversation and then she asked me who had 'ghosted' a recent article that I had written for the *Guardian* women's page. I looked at her blankly: 'Ghosted?' I said. 'I'm not sure what you mean. I wrote it myself.' Lady Collins raised an eyebrow and by the end of the interview I had agreed to write a book for Collins for an advance of five thousand pounds: fifteen hundred pounds on signing, fifteen hundred on delivery of manuscript and two thousand on publication. It was six times what Penguin had offered me and it felt like a small fortune.

So it was that I began to write my first book and discovered that I really enjoyed writing. For me, writing has always been fairly simple: I begin at the beginning and tell my story, reflect along the way and finish it. I am not one of those writers who produce draft after draft – no doubt I'd be better if I did! I write about thirty pages of hand script a day, correct it at the end of the day and once again in the morning, then get it typed and read it again. My first book, *Audacity to Believe*, was written in dribs and drabs, in between lectures and TV engagements. Before I went away, I'd be so terrified of being burgled by the Chilean Secret Police that I would hide the manuscript – usually at the bottom of the laundry basket. By the time I returned a week or so later, I'd have forgotten where I'd hidden it and would wail that the DINA had discovered it and carried it off to Chile!

The fear of repercussions from Chile was never far away. In London, if a taxi turned down a side street, my heart turned over and I would expect the men in dark glasses to appear from nowhere. The fact that my fears were probably unfounded made little difference: fear is fear whether there is a valid reason for it or not. In fact, it was very difficult to know whether or not I was in danger. The Chilean refugees were convinced that there were spies in their midst and in 1976, Orlando Letelier, an exiled Chilean politician, was assassinated outside his home in Washington. The fact that I had had breakfast with Orlando and his family a week before he was killed brought home to me the reality of the DINA abroad in a particularly unpleasant way.

It has emerged, over the years, that there was a network of security forces throughout Latin America named Operation Condor, through which serious 'troublemakers' were tracked down and 'eliminated'. Letelier was one of their victims, ex-General Arturo Prats (killed in Argentina) another, as was Bernado Leighton who was seriously injured during an attack in Rome. I remember that when I was anxious about visiting the USA, a friend rang up the Foreign Office to see if I was at any risk. The answer was chilling, 'No more than she is in this country.'

After a while, the pressure of so much public exposure began to tell and I had difficulty sleeping. I would either not be able to sleep at night or wake very early in the morning. This was particularly stressful as my talks were all given without notes and, the more tired I was, the more I worried that I would dry up, forget what to say and make a fool of myself. This insomnia was to plague me off and on for the next seventeen years and was, for me, the bitterest legacy of my Chilean adventure. With hindsight, I think this was a manifestation of post-traumatic stress disorder which became a chronic state. I have endless diary entries that read: 'It is 2 a.m. I still cannot sleep. My heart pounds', and so on. I would sit and weep in self-pity and worry desperately about the following day. It was not, however, until many years later that I sought help from a psychiatrist and then from a psychotherapist. Even after nearly ten years of psychotherapy I still had difficulty sleeping and it wasn't until I was given antidepressants that my anxiety disappeared and I was able to go to bed confident that I would sleep. I have remained on this medication since 1992 and see no reason to stop it.

In August of 1976, at the suggestion of my Jesuit advisor, Father Paul Kennedy, I spent two weeks inside the cloister of Stanbrook Abbey, an enclosed Benedictine monastery for women. It was a rare privilege extended to me by the nuns and provided me with space to pray and reflect upon what I was doing. I remember being entranced by the plainchant, especially Compline sung from memory in a darkened church. It was a large community and the standard of the singing was very high. I had thought that I would miss the outside world terribly but there was a curious feeling of one-upmanship being inside and shutting the rest of the world out. I would sit in the garden for hours looking at a fallen leaf and marvelling that it contained, in miniature, all the beauty of the universe. It was a particularly hot summer and one of the nuns would cut the dead heads off the roses. I would look at these shrivelled corpses and somehow see in them the precious lives cut off in the Chilean conflict.

There were a couple of young aspirants there at the same time, women 'trying' their vocation to the monastic life. One of them left while I was there and I watched from my bedroom window as her family collected her. Her mother had brought a large Tupperware box of cakes or some goodies and I saw her tuck into these eagerly as the car turned to leave. It wasn't that we didn't have enough to eat, but our fare was very plain. I can't remember what we had for breakfast, but whatever it was I thought it wasn't enough and I sent the nuns a sackful of muesli after I left! My generosity paid off because they changed their breakfast menu shortly after. My two weeks 'inside' at Stanbrook was enough to persuade me that I didn't belong there, but it was many years before I could let go of the conviction that I had a calling to the monastic life.

Sometime that same August I was invited to speak at a human rights conference hosted by the Catholic Church at the headquarters of the Maryknoll missionaries at Ossining, outside New York. It was a very happy adventure for I felt deeply at home among the Maryknoll sisters.

These were nuns unlike any others I had met: brave, pragmatic women with a powerful sense of call to spread the Gospel. I was immediately welcomed as part of the Latin American community and spent many happy mealtimes meeting women who worked in Chile, Brazil or other countries. What I liked about the Maryknollers was their lack of fuss: one day I'd have coffee with Mary or Beth or Ellen and the next day her chair would be empty. 'Oh, she's gone back to Brazil,' someone would say: 'she left at six this morning. We didn't like to wake you!'

After the conference I made a brief trip to Washington to speak and appear on TV, and then it was back to the UK. It was on this occasion that I met Orlando Letelier who was so tragically assassinated a week later. The opportunity to meet with a number of radical church people was a powerful spur to keep up my human rights work.

Sister Connie Kelly who had been in the house when I was arrested was back in New York and Pat and I stayed with her and three fellow sisters in their house in the Bronx. It was quite an eye-opener to try to sleep in a humid tenement building with music and noise from the street which went on all night. Eventually, I dragged my mattress into the bathroom and slept on the floor, wedged in by the bath. It was hard to reconcile my image of myself as a fearless human rights activist with my personal need for regular meals and creature comforts!

Once back in the UK, I continued my rackety life of public speaking and fitted in the writing as best I could. In October, I was due to speak at a human rights day service in Leeds, but I was recovering from a chest infection so read the lesson instead. From there I went to stay in the guest house at Ampleforth Abbey, a large Benedictine monastery for men, to correct the proofs of my book. I can't believe now that I wrote *Audacity to Believe* in about six months, but I know the proofs were ready for correction that October. There was also a note from my editor, saying that the book was so long that, not only would nobody be able to afford it, they wouldn't be able to lift it! So I spent the next two weeks editing it. At the beginning it seemed an impossible task, but, as the days went by and I slept ever more poorly, I became bored with my own handi-work and was able to take a blue crayon to the required 25 per cent of the manuscript.

Sometime after this, I received a letter from one of the nuns of the Religious of the Sacred Heart asking if I was still serious about joining their congregation. (I had sent a formal letter requesting admission after making a retreat in Chile.) Had I ever really meant to join them? I'm not sure. I was certainly determined to give my life to God, but, the truth is, I always wanted to be a monk rather than a nun. This reminder of my Malloco commitment came as a nasty shock at the height of my public life, but, determined not to go back on my word, I went to visit them at their large college at Roehampton. They were extremely courteous and I was shown round the college and where the nuns lived. As we walked around the science block, the Principal, who was showing me round, mentioned casually that I would be able to teach botany. This shook me to my roots, for although I knew that entering the convent meant giving up my own will and doing what I was told, it had never dawned on me that I would not continue in the practice of medicine! The worst moment, however, was when I saw the nuns' rooms. There was a black hospital-style bed with a pale green cover and nothing much else. No divan, no pictures. I could have burst into tears and howled, as I had done in Oslo: 'This is worse than bloody prison!' I held my tongue, however, and went on to be interviewed by the formation team, the sisters in charge of women newly joining the order. I don't quite know what it was, but I felt supremely ill at ease. They were so tidy, so controlled and *so* intelligent. It didn't help me to make a good impression when I had to lie down on the floor during the interview because my back hurt so much!

After a while, they suggested that perhaps I might spend three months without any public engagements before I entered. Once again, I felt a sense of outrage: did they not know, these women, that I was a latter-day Joan of Arc, single-handedly engaged in my God-given mission to rescue the political prisoners of Chile? Did they not *care*? I thought to myself. But I said nothing, and we fixed a date for me to enter: 25 March, the Feast of the Annunciation. I left them, thankfully, and returned to Devon to begin my preparation for religious life.?

I write all this slightly tongue in cheek, because thirty years on I can stand back and see how crazy I was ever to think I could survive in a convent. I am an extremely idiosyncratic woman, brought up largely in the company of men (in the 1950s and 60s men far outnumbered women in medicine) and I do not take kindly to melting into the group. I am also highly creative and seriously messy with it, so I am a nightmare in any communal space.

After Christmas, I went back to Ampleforth to give a lecture on human rights to the sixth-formers. This proved to be a key visit, for I became friendly with Father Tom Cullinan, one of the monks, and we swapped visions of modern monastic life. Tom, and two other monks, David and Aidan, were planning to start a new and radically simple monastic foundation and I found their ideas enormously exciting. While in Chile,

I used to go every six weeks for a long weekend in a house of prayer by the sea. It was run by two Maryknoll sisters who felt a calling to the contemplative life and provided hospitality for those who needed time and space out of their missionary lives. They rose at four and prayed in silence. I used to join them and prayed lying face down on the floor in an act of adoration, interrupted only by occasional falling asleep and being woken by my own snoring.

I loved my time there and developed a vision of a similar way of life in which a small core of monastic men and women would live together and provide an escape and hospitality for the workers in the 'marketplace': priests, teachers, doctors and so on who have so little opportunity to pray or just 'be'.

My conversations with Tom re-awakened these ideas and I wrote out an account of my 'vision'. Tom showed it to the Abbot and, within twenty-four hours, I was offered a cottage on the Ampleforth school campus to experiment in creating a new model of monastic life for women. The next eighteen months, living in the shadow of the monastery and gently flirting with the monks, was one of the happiest times of my life and, had they allowed me, I think I'd have stayed there for ever.

18

PLAYING MONKS:
1977

Whe n Abbot Ambrose said that I could come to Ampleforth for three months to explore my vision, something shifted inside me. It was like fiddling with a combination lock: suddenly there was a click, things fell into place and I knew what I had to do. A cynic might say that I had found a spiritually plausible excuse for getting out of entering the convent and that could well be true. No matter. I was full of resolve and laid my plans swiftly. I returned to Devon and within a month was back as the mistress of St Laurence's Cottage at Ampleforth, about five minutes' walk from the abbey church. The hope was that, with the help of the monks, I would evolve a modern way of religious life and would be joined by other young women with similar aspirations.

As I set out to work out my order of day I was clear on one thing: prayer should be central. This was for me the key difference between the monastic and the 'active' religious life. In the 'active' orders the work seemed to be primary and prayer was, as it were, fitted into the cracks. My understanding of monastic life was that the Divine Office (psalms and readings) was the framework, the core of the life, and it was the work which was fitted into the interstices. So it was that I went down to the abbey church to pray with the monks five times a day: for Matins at 6.00 a.m., Lauds and Mass at 7.10 a.m., Midday Office at 1.10 p.m., Vespers at 7.00 p.m. and Compline at 9.00 p.m. I found the rhythm of the day and the liturgical seasons magical. Although rising in the dark of winter and walking down a steep hill to the abbey was tough, and the monotone of this first office of the day unappealing, there was something enormously fortifying about being in a group of people all doing something as crazy as singing hymns before the sun was up. I will readily admit that I was seeing the life through rose-tinted spectacles but, even now, if I slip into the choir stalls and listen to the familiar cadence of the Gregorian chant, I am filled with a deep sense of calm and joy.

The monks were very patient with me, because they were not all happy to be seen by outsiders so early in the day, particularly by an over-chirpy middle-aged woman. As the aim of my presence at the monastery was to learn about the monastic life and listen to any call which God might be making of me, I was assigned tutors in the key subjects of Scripture and monastic spirituality and I was allowed to join some of the junior monks for theology classes. Of all the things in my life for which I am grateful, I think my introduction to the Scriptures is one of the most important. My tutor was Father Bonaventure Knollys, a shy monk with a wide knowledge and a deep love of the Bible. He introduced me to the 'annotated' Jerusalem Bible and showed me how to trace themes between the Old and New Testaments. At first, I found it terribly difficult to understand the Scriptures. My schooling hitherto had been in the sciences and I found the use of myth and imagery tiresome and alien. Little by little, however, I learned to read the texts less literally and then, to my surprise, I saw the meaning more clearly. Reading the Bible is a journey and one needs a companion who knows the way; studying the Old Testament in particular is a bit like panning for gold or searching for precious stones in granite: the magic passages suddenly glint at you, and when they do, you are dazzled. Most of all, I love Isaiah, particularly the famous advent passage in chapter 9, so familiar to all who love *The Messiah*:

> The people that walked in darkness
> has seen a great light;
> on those who live in a land of deep shadow
> a light has shone.
>
> For there is a child born for us,
> a son given to us
> and dominion is laid on his shoulders;
> and this is the name they give him:
> Wonder-Counsellor, Mighty-God,
> Eternal-Father, Prince-of-Peace. (Isaiah 9:1, 5)

I think that the Old Testament works for me because I have always been more 'theocentric' than I have been 'christocentric'. By this I mean that, although I value the gospels and the Christian story, I find far more sense of the Divine in the more mythical language of the Old Testament. Isaiah, in particular, 'turns me on' spiritually – fills me with a sense of awe and wonder and love in a way that the Jesus stories never have. It is not so much a matter of theology as one of personal idiosyncrasy: I have more sense of God transcendent than I have of God incarnate. Job, too, is another favourite, particularly the last three chapters in which God speaks to Job from the heart of the tempest:

> Where were you when I laid the earth's foundations?
>   Tell me, since you are so well-informed!
> Who decided the dimensions of it, do you know?
>
> Who pent up the sea behind closed doors
>   when it leapt tumultuous out of the womb,
> when I wrapped it in a robe of mist
>   and made black clouds its swaddling bands;
> when I marked the bounds it was not to cross
>   and made it fast with a bolted gate?
> Come thus far, I said, and no farther:
>   here your proud waves shall break. (Job 38:4–5, 8–11)

My three years of monastic living, with its regular diet of psalms and Old and New Testament, has given me a familiarity with the Scriptures which I don't think I could have achieved in any other way. It has also given me a foundation knowledge which has enabled me to continue linking scriptural truths with daily living. It is from this foundation that I have been able to do a considerable amount of religious broadcasting and preaching over the past twenty-five years or so. For the past seventeen years I have also done some scriptural commentaries for daily reading for the International Bible Reading Association and for CAFOD (Catholic Action for Overseas Development), a labour which enables me to share my excitement over my favourite passages and also to reflect upon parts which are unfamiliar.

My other major study at Ampleforth was monastic history and spirituality. Father Bernard Green, then Brother Bernard, was an enthralling teacher with an amazing broad knowledge of the development of Christianity and in particular of monastic history. He explained to me, in particular, the difference between the *cataphatic* and *apophatic* schools of spirituality. Although this sounds very technical, I have actually found it enormously helpful in understanding my own way to God and that of other people. The *cataphatic* way speaks of God's attributes: he is good, and just, merciful and slow to anger. It is a comforting way because it gives us a notion of God that we can grasp: a God who was made manifest in the man Jesus. The *apophatic* way, if I understand it right, is based on a sense of God as mystery, or the belief that we can never *know* God, that is, although we may know about his *works*, it is beyond our human capacity to understand him (or her). The person following this way will not say God is this or God is that, but quite simply that *God IS*. It is difficult to explain the frissons of awe and wonder that this simple phrase produces in me. It is also impossible to explain how someone can have a personal relationship with this unknown and unknowable God. Father Cyprian Smith, another monk of Ampleforth, writes about the God of Paradox: God who is unknowable, and yet we 'know' him carnally, as a woman 'knows' a man. This kind of language is trying to describe the indescribable: trying to capture what is called the *immanence*, the closeness, and *transcendence*, the otherness, of God. God is transcendent: infinitely different from us, beyond the furthest star; and yet he is immanent – as the prophet Muhammad put it, 'as near as the neck of my camel'. This is, of course, the language of the mystics, but it is a language which makes total sense to some quite ordinary people, including me.

One of the things which has always fascinated and enthralled me is to trace the way this spirituality of the mystery of God has developed and been preserved among successive groups of people, relatively apart from the more mainstream Christian faith. I am *not* saying that the apophatic way is not Christian; rather, that it has perhaps a greater awareness of the mysterious risen Christ than the Jesus of history. I have to admit to finding mildly irritating the widespread tendency to use the words 'Jesus' and 'Christ' interchangeably. As St Paul writes, 'Christ is the image of the unseen God, the first born of all creation', while Jesus was God incarnate, God made human like us, like you, like me. Jesus lived in Palestine, two thousand odd years ago, and he died, so we are told, in AD 33. Christ is God – alive now and for ever.

I find this distinction important because by confusing the historical Jesus with the risen Christ, we have a very anthropomorphic notion of God, that is, we think of God as Jesus the man, and lose sight of the wild, mysterious nature of our Creator. It is not that Jesus was a good, kind man and therefore God must be like that, but that the unseen God of the Old Testament loves his people with an amazing passion – a notion that the mystics try to convey in passages like the Song of Songs. The jealous lover whom we meet in the 'Hound of Heaven' is very different from the image of the song-writer who wrote 'What a friend we have in Jesus'. As Tony de Mello, the Indian Jesuit psychologist, wrote: 'Empty out your tea-cup God!' – your notion of God is too small, too limiting, too confining.

Of course, there always has been, and no doubt there always will be, a degree of conflict between those who follow the way of the God of Mystery and those who need a more human-shaped God. If what Bernard told me is right, some of the early Desert Fathers had a notion that God was like themselves, only bigger. They were, therefore, very distressed when Evagrius, a Greek-trained theologian, tried to debunk their vision of God. 'You have taken away my God,' they cried and wept bitter tears.

I remember vividly how lost I felt when my own anthropomorphic God image failed me. It was following a conversation with the Australian monk Father Placid Spearitt, now Prior of the monastery of New Norcia in Western Australia. Placid is a devotee of the German mystics, particularly Meister Eckhart and Ruysbroeck, and of the seventeenth-century English Benedictine Augustine Baker. It was Augustine Baker who taught the Benedictine nuns of Stanbrook (then at Cambrai, in France) this way, and he has also greatly influenced the spirituality of the monks of the English Benedictine Congregation, that is, the men of Downside, Ampleforth, Douay and Belmont.

The Old Testament, particularly Isaiah, presents a very paradoxical notion of the Divine: the God who emerges is the creator of light and darkness, the author of good and evil, harsh judge and tender lover, separately and all at once. It is not of course that God is this or that, but that the authors of the book of Isaiah, like those before and after them, are struggling to make sense of the world in which they live: a world of stunning beauty and terrible pain: a world of mystery.

The Alexandrian Jew, Philo, who lived at the same time as Jesus, wrote of the way we search for God but never find him, but are somehow satisfied in the searching. Following him was Evagrius, one of the early desert scholars, who was well versed in the studies of the Greek philosophers. Evagrius taught widely in the desert and indirectly influenced many people including the Cappadocians, St Gregory of Nyssa and Gregory Nazianzen. Then, from Syria, we have the mysterious figure of Dionysius whose writings were revered for centuries. These writings were sent as a gift from the Bishop of Constantinople to the French king and from there they entered the mainstream of German culture and had a wide influence on the Rhineland scholars, from whose schools we get Eckhart, Ruysbroeck and Tauler.

The main source of inspiration, however, came in a little book by an unknown British monk, *The Cloud of Unknowing*. This work was much read by the recusant monks and nuns: by those men and women who had entered religious life in English monasteries located in France because of the persecution of Catholics in the UK. The author of the *Cloud* (for he is never named) writes a letter of instruction for a young disciple in which he tells him to avoid all images of God and all pious discourse, setting heart and mind to penetrate, in all simplicity, that mysterious barrier, that metaphorical 'cloud of unknowing' in which God is to be found. He tells his followers to pierce the cloud with little darts of love and longing, using no more than one word. Some interpreters take this for an instruction to use a mantra, a word used repetitively to still the mind. My own experience of using a mantra in meditation, however, has been one of discord; I find that complete silence or centring using observation of the breath more conducive to inner silence. It is, I believe, a matter of taste or personal idiosyncrasy.

Alongside the apophatic way there has grown the more commonly accepted Christian spirituality in which Jesus is loved as a personal friend. This spirituality is much more Gospel-based and is less at home in the wilder reaches of Isaiah or the Song of Songs. When I was a child and a young woman, Catholics were brought up on the gospels and St Paul and were not encouraged to read the Hebrew Scriptures. Perhaps this is why generations of Catholics are more at home in a Jesus-centred spirituality and are suspicious of modern meditation techniques.

My guess is that it doesn't really matter how we pray so long as we enter into a living relationship with God. The danger, however, with a naive and unthinking acceptance of too simple an interpretation of Christianity is that it may not stand up in times of crisis. If we believe in a loving Daddy (Abba) God who will give us what we want provided we ask, then we are likely to be both disappointed and disillusioned if God does not come to our rescue if we are sick or otherwise in trouble. This is an age-old problem of the devout: we have only to read some of the psalms which promise that God will reward the just and punish the wicked. It is enormously comforting but it just doesn't work if your child is raped or murdered and the killer is never caught.

It seems to me important to state this clearly, because as a doctor whose work plunges me constantly into the pain of others, I meet many people who discard their religion as a useless fantasy in time of trouble. And this is not their fault. If they have been brought up to believe in a Santa Claus God who will look after his followers then they are bound to be desperately disillusioned. That is why I find the God of mystery the only God who makes sense to me. Isaiah's God who makes both darkness and light, joy and pain, life and death is the only God I can believe in. Of course, I don't understand this God: he, she, is infinitely beyond my capacity to understand, but I am deeply content to live in unknowing.

This is where the prayer of silence and emptiness is so helpful, for it is in this silence and unknowing that I 'meet' God and know myself loved. Once you know in your guts that you are loved then you can dare to trust. I write these particular pages on holiday in Lanzarote where I am educated each day by my great nephew Harry who, at three and a half, is meeting the world through unbiased eyes. Yesterday, in the sea, he clung like a limpet to the back of his mother Lucy while she swam. He trusted her, but only so far, because each time she set out for the deep he would wail and demand to be set ashore. We are a bit like Harry: we only trust God so far, but no further. If we want to have a wider view of life, however, we must be brave. We went to see the Lanzarote volcanoes and, after driving round the amazing, bleak landscape with its mountains and craters, we had the opportunity to ride on a camel. At first we were scared, but, taking our courage in our hands, we climbed onto the wooden frames and were tied in with a piece of rope. All was well while we sat there with the camel at rest, but then the time came for it to rise and we were hoisted into the air, losing all personal control of the situation. At first, I felt sick with fear, but after a few yards I relaxed and understood what an amazing experience it was. We walked along the narrow paths up the mountain, and enjoyed the stunning views around us. The camels went nose to tail, led up the desert tracks. Perhaps this can be an image for the way of unknowing: the landscape is bleak but wondrously beautiful. One is led, quite out of control, but if one relaxes, the movement becomes familiar and delightful and it seems perfectly sensible to trust.

My friend, Maryknoll Sister Carla Piette, who drowned in El Salvador, once wrote while on retreat: 'I feel as if I'm on a taxi ride and I don't know where I'm going, but it's OK because I trust the Cabbie.' God as Cabbie, Camel Driver, Lover: there is no end to the imagery because our relationships with the Divine are each unique and we can only ever struggle for words to describe our experience.

*

After I had been at Ampleforth for three months, Abbot Ambrose extended my permission to stay to eighteen months. So, for a year and a half I attended the Divine Office, listened to the Scriptures and became 'pickled' in the psalms as all monks do. I did not, however, experience community life: that was to come later. I paid for my accommodation and tuition by a little work: I cooked supper at the Grange, the retreat house, on a Monday evening and did a couple of hours of photocopying and cyclostyling each afternoon. I also arranged the flowers in the church and had great adventures stealing azaleas from the woods on the edge of the monastery land where there are three small lakes surrounded by trees and bushes.

After a few months, I became more or less accepted by the monks, although those who resented my presence were far too polite to say so. I remember the day I left for good, one of my friends said, 'Oh, Father X was asking if you'd gone.'

'Oh,' I said, cheerily, 'I'll go and say goodbye.'

'No, I wouldn't,' he said. 'He was just asking if you'd gone!'

I spent a lot of time and mental energy during my sojourn at Ampleforth trying to work out what the monastic life was *for*. Each time I thought I had it sussed, I'd say to Bonaventure, 'Now I understand! It's for this or that . . .' Bon would grin and say, 'It's not *for* anything. It just *is*.' I suspect he was right. Such a way of life makes no sense in human terms: it's just what some people get drawn to do because that's where their relationship with God – their camel ride – takes them. Placid used to say, 'You shouldn't join a monastery unless you absolutely *have* to.' I never asked him to expand, but I think I know what he means.

Quite early in my stay, I was joined by a woman who simply *had* to be a monk, or rather a nun. I found she was very different from me, which is hardly surprising, but I didn't understand then that I didn't really have a calling to the monastic life. Jane (which is not her real name) had been a ballet dancer and was a convert to Catholicism. She'd already spent eighteen months in a convent but had not been happy and had left. She was a highly disciplined woman with a hunger for God quite different from mine. She stayed with me three months and then re-entered several other convents until she eventually decided to live her life as a solitary, although in the 'ordinary' world. Of the other young women who came to discuss their difficulties in finding a religious life that met their needs, one tried her vocation in another Benedictine convent but left after five years to return to medical practice, although she now lives as a solitary near a large monastery in Germany. Another, Ann, who had been a

Carmelite nun but had had to leave because of illness returned to another Carmel and has been happily settled there for the past twenty years. Another entered the Franciscans but left and has not been in contact. Two older sisters, one Dominican and one Benedictine, have both elected to live their lives as religious but outside the cloister.

In my Ampleforth days, I was so sure that I knew what the religious life was about and was only too ready to hold forth or give advice. Now, thirty years on, I have no such pretensions, though I retain a fascination with the notion of abandoning all in the service of God. These days, however, my understanding of Christianity is much simpler and can be summed up in the words of St John the Evangelist when he says, 'Anyone who says I love God and hates his brother is a liar, since a man who does not love the brother that he can see cannot love God whom he has never seen. So this is the commandment that he has given us, that anyone who loves God must also love his brother' (1 John 4:20–21).

As the eighteen months of my time at Ampleforth came to an end, in consultation with a few advisers, I decided that the next step was to undertake a novitiate (a period of prayer and training) in a suitable monastic house for women. My friend Father Barnabas Sandeman, one of the older monks of the Ampleforth community and adviser to many enclosed convents, suggested that I should spend time with the Bernadine sisters in Slough, a group of Cistercian women who had their roots in Belgium after religious life had been banned in England. These nuns differed from the Benedictines (who took a vow of stability in a particular monastery) in that their allegiance was to a worldwide community of women who moved as appropriate between their houses.

In October of 1978, therefore, I packed up my belongings and took myself off to St Bernard's Convent in Slough where I entered as a 'postulant' at the age of forty-two. I was full of hope and enthusiasm although secretly afraid that this was God's devious way of getting me into a convent. My plan was to complete the novitiate experience and then, if my vision still seemed valid, to begin a small monastic community which would be true to the essentials of monastic life but free of the centuries-old accretions which have made the lives of nuns so different from those of their male counterparts.

19

PLAYING NUNS –
THE REAL McCOY:
NOVEMBER 1978

S t Bernard's Convent in Slough is home to the Bernardines, a
monastic order based on the rule of St Bernard of Clairvaux, the
twelfth-century founder of the Cistercians, better known as the
Trappists. The friends who know me now fall about laughing and
ask what on earth persuaded me that I could survive in an enclosed
convent where silence was part of the rule. The fact is that I *didn't* know
if the decision was right, and, indeed, it turned out to be wrong, for I was
asked to leave eighteen months later because I was so unhappy. It is
important to emphasise, however, that I have never regretted having
entered: I *had* to do it, to find out once and for always whether I had a
'vocation', whether God was calling me to be a nun.

After I left Ampleforth, for the month before I entered the convent, I
went to stay with three friends, monks of Ampleforth, who were living a
simplified form of monastic life outside Liverpool. The idea was that this
would be a combination holiday and pre-novitiate, to give my friends a
chance to warn me of any little ways I had which might be detrimental to
my settling into a community. It was a happy month and I am deeply
grateful to them.

The little monastery of Ince Benet, on the Southport road, was for
many years very dear to my heart. It was started by three monks, Thomas,
David and Aidan, who, feeling uncomfortable about the prosperity and

complexity of Ampleforth, moved out in 1978 to start afresh, just as in the eleventh century St Bernard moved out of the great monastery at Cluny to start again more simply at Clairvaux. There is a great deal to be said for starting again: I calculate that I have done it five times myself! The three monks had, initially, wanted to begin in one of the inner-city areas of Liverpool but were advised by those who already lived there that they would be more use to everyone if they were at one remove. They began, therefore, in a borrowed house on a large private estate near Crosby. Right from the beginning, they were determined to live as simply as possible: they had no fridge, no telephone and no washing machine, and, amazingly, thirty years later they manage without what most of us see as necessities of life. The fact is, if you grow your own vegetables, use powdered milk and do your washing a little at a time, it is perfectly possible to live in this way.

This month at Ince Benet was very important to me, for the monks were living out a masculine version of the vision that I had developed, quite unaware of their thinking. (I'm sure, however, that I would have had a fridge, phone and washing machine!) The Divine Office was, of course, central to the structure of the day. The monks wore a cowl (a long black robe) over jeans or shorts and sat cross legged on the floor. The melodies were adapted for just a few voices and although it never had, for me, the magic of the full Gregorian chant, it was very lovely.

The monks' aim was to develop a way of monastic living which would be painfully aware of the injustice and suffering of the world. It was also to be in contact with the poor of this country and they would model a style of living which cost little in financial terms. There is a sense, of course, in which the British poor *could* live a simple life like the monks, without phone, TV or fridge, but tastes and needs are different and it is one thing to *choose* to be poor, quite another to have poverty thrust upon you. Life is always so much more complicated in practice than it is in theory.

Ince Benet continues up to the time of writing, although Tom has been on his own for many years. As so often happens, a venture which was planned to develop in one way has grown quite differently. Three of the monks who joined him in the early days have moved on, and Father Barnabas Sandeman, one of the very senior monks at Ampleforth, sadly died of a heart attack not long after joining. One of my happiest memories is teaching him how to make onion soup: a delightful exchange of tuition! Although Barnabas had been a monk of Ampleforth since he was a young man, he was deliciously young at heart. He was extremely enthusiastic about the Ince Benet vision and very supportive of me in my efforts to prepare myself for a radically new way of life. He himself had written an article questioning the future of monastic life in the twenty-first century. It was entitled 'Solomon's Temple or Abraham's Tent' and compared the old-established monasteries which had such difficulty adapting to change with the simplicity of the new vision which could pack up and move its tent on without major upset and discord.

I am well aware of the difficulty of implementing any change in monastic life. In any community there is usually a wide span of ages, from the very old to the new comers. In Benedictine communities which are stable, that is, where the members do not move about between monasteries, it is inevitable that those in their forties and fifties who are involved in policy-making must consider the views of the elderly who will almost certainly include their former superiors, the prioresses and novice mistresses. The monastic set-up is a bit like a very large extended family. So long as our mother is alive, it is difficult to implement change: and, of course, elderly nuns can live to great ages. There is, understandably, great respect for the older members of the family and much care is taken not to upset them. The problem is that the 'young radicals' are well into late middle age before the ancestors die, and by this time they themselves are set in their ways and in no mood to accept suggestions from the latest batch of pushy 'adolescents'. It may well be that monastic life as it is today is too entrenched to change and that new life, in the form of informal communities, will spring up. Having said that, it is the numbers in the apostolic orders that are diminishing and the monastic orders are still relatively strong. The Holy Spirit no doubt has her own views, but she's not telling!

Eventually, I had to stop playing monks, which had been such a happy game for nearly two years, and steel myself to try out life in a real convent. So, on 1 November, the anniversary of my imprisonment, I willingly submitted myself to the 'yoke' of obedience as an aspirant in a convent in darkest Slough. I came travelling light (by my standards, I hasten to add!). I brought all my theology and Scripture books, explaining that, of course, they were for everyone's use, far too many clothes and a selection of pens, boots and other survival items. I remember the last night frantically sewing a little Peruvian woolly rug onto the outside of a bag as a surreptitious comfort object. (If I had to enter a convent now, I don't think I'd be prepared to go without my teddy bear! If ever a woman needed a bear, it is in a convent for they are singularly comfortless places.)

I was given a room with the rest of the community in what I think had once been a dormitory and a desk in the novices' *scriptorium* or writing room. I should explain that the Cistercians, whose rule the nuns followed, believed in the discipline of life in community, that is, the monks did not have study bedrooms of their own but slept in a dormitory and worked together. I found working in the scriptorium both friendly and hard. We were given children's school desks with a lift-up lid and, as someone used to occupying whole houses with my papers, I went nearly mad with frustration. No sooner had I arranged my papers on the sloping surface than I needed something from inside the desk and would try to hold things in place with one hand while scrabbling in the mess inside for whatever I wanted. After I'd been there a few months my two fellow novices took pity on me and found a six-foot folding table which they moved into the novitiate for me. I felt as though Christmas had come and arranged my things with great delight. The novice mistress was not amused but she let me keep it.

This was really the story of my life in the monastery: I was always finding ways of defeating the system and felt hurt when I was rebuked. The trouble is I don't really like conforming to anyone else's laws and have never seen the virtue in being one of the crowd. I am, it seems, by nature an individualist and, as such, simply could not conform to convent life. It was the custom to start the day's worship at 6.30 a.m. in the chapel: but I always had to be there earlier, not for the sake of being different, but because I couldn't see any reason to conform. I always pray more easily and ardently on my own and on my early morning jaunts I would sit on the floor at the back of the chapel and delight in the empty space, which always gives me a sense of the Divine. Alas, even this simple spiritual pleasure upset people, for my leaning against the wall left a mark and the elderly sister whose job it was to keep the chapel spotless in the Lord's honour complained to the novice mistress who told me that, if I *had* to pray at a different time to the rest of the community, would I please kneel or sit in a pew like anyone else. I was secretly humiliated yet again. The trouble was my knees hurt when I kneel down and my back hurts when I sit in an ill-designed pew and I don't feel at all devout! I thank God that nowadays I can share my early morning tea with my Maker and no one can complain that it is irreverent and dissolute to pray like this.

There were good times too and I greatly enjoyed the regular life. I liked rising early, and I particularly liked being fed on time! The food in the convent was good and plentiful and I found it very satisfactory being read to during meals because it meant I didn't have to make polite conversation with anyone. I enjoyed the intellectual work enormously and embarked upon a self-chosen study of the origins of humanity from a marvellous text book which I found before I entered. It was really exciting to read about the way civilization began in Mesopotamia and in the Nile Delta, though I don't think my novice mistress was particularly enthusiastic. With hindsight, I see that I was filling the emptiness of my life with study: not, I suspect, an uncommon sublimation technique. The worst part of each day was the time reserved for 'recreation' and I found it seriously stressful. There were two half-hours, one after lunch and one after supper, when the community came together to do hand work and to chat. Alas, in those days I didn't know how to knit and I was both bored and anxious. With hindsight, I think it was because I have very little small talk and was not yet mature (or generous) enough to try to entertain the others. The novice mistress did point this out to the three of us novices when we muttered about how boring it was, but we weren't in a mood to concede the battle. When I described the situation to my sister-in-law she grinned and said, 'It sounds like a cocktail party without the booze!', which was the most accurate description I've heard yet. I think the main problem was the name of this ceremony: had I been told that it was a penitential service I would no doubt have taken it in my stride, but I thought it was supposed to be fun and found it a dismal failure.

One of the main duties of the novices was housework, the novitiate year being designed to give us an experience of the routine of monastic life without too much excitement or disruption. I have never liked house-work and, because of this, am extremely bad at it. Having for many years hired people to clean my home I did not find the tasks of dusting, lavatory cleaning and polishing an attractive prospect and was quick witted enough to raise, in all humility, of course, the problem of my asthma. Like most asthmatics, I am allergic to dust, so the novice mistress sighed and set me to clean windows, which I quite enjoyed. My favourite manual labour, however, was working in the garden and I became the devoted disciple of a delightful elderly sister who taught me the ways of Mother Earth. In the autumn of my second year I discovered the joys of leaf raking and bonfires and spent evening after evening with the headmistress of the school, herself a nun. Together we raked the leaves and made damp smoky fires, which did far more harm to my lungs than a little gentle dusting would ever have done. It turned out that I was also allergic to leaf mould and my asthma flared up dramatically. My own doctor, or rather the doctor of my medical student days, lived in Oxford so I refused to be registered with the nuns' GP and took myself off to

Oxford to see him. He, fearing that the monastic life was too hard for me, put me into the isolation hospital in Oxford where I had a happy period of respite from the rigours of the convent.

The best thing about being a monk (I could never bear to think of myself as a nun) was the liturgy, by which I mean the daily arrangement of the psalms, Scripture and hymns, which together make up what is called the Divine Office. It is difficult to explain how, when one is starved of TV, theatre and virtually all aesthetic input, the poetry of Isaiah and the sound of good voices singing can thrill the heart. One of my great sadnesses in the convent was the fact that I had difficulty singing the office. Although I have a powerful speaking voice, my singing is extremely erratic: sometimes my voice seems to work, but mostly it doesn't and I am much more at home singing with male voices than with female ones.

By March of 1980 I was relatively settled in the convent and determined to stick it out until the two years which I had set myself were complete. As I explained at the end of the last chapter, when I entered the convent I had no intention of staying longer than two years. I saw my time there as the traditional two-year monastic novitiate which, as founder of a new form of monastic life, I would be obliged to undertake. I did, however, leave space in my mind and heart for this to be God's crafty way of getting me into a convent. What the nuns felt, I've no idea, but my guess is they knew I was not monk 'material'. That this was truly the case was soon to be demonstrated when my Chilean past caught up with me with a vengeance.

20

I LEAVE THE CONVENT: MARCH 1980

O ne morning in March 1980 something happened which turned my tranquil world as a novice upside down: the Chilean drama, quiescent for over four years, suddenly flared up again. It happened like this: I was sent a copy of a letter to *The Times* commenting on a current debate about whether or not Britain should restore diplomatic relations with Chile. The writer said that it was high time relations were restored so that business could resume and that there was far too much nonsense talked about human rights abuses; or something to that effect. The Chile Committee requested me to write a letter to *The Times* in reply, so, not seeing why I shouldn't, I wrote a spirited reply mentioning the recent discovery of a mass grave containing three hundred bodies. Knowing that the novice mistress would not approve of this very public communication with the outside world, I gave it to a friend to post and omitted to inform her of what I had done. The letter was duly published in *The Times* with a rather dramatic typographical error which increased the number of bodies found from three hundred to three thousand! I thought no more about it until a week or so later I received an extremely unpleasant 'poison pen' letter saying, 'We'll get you, you Marxist whore', or words to that effect. Hate mail is always unpleasant but I found this one particularly scary as it was written in an educated hand. I took it to the prioress, a very intelligent woman, for whom I had great respect, and she locked it away.

With hindsight, I've often wondered if the events which were to follow could be in any way related to that letter. Who can tell? A week or so after

I received the letter, I was making my way from the chapel to the dining room for breakfast. My route took me past the headmistress's door and she beckoned me in and handed me the morning paper, saying something like, 'You need to know about this'. On the front page of one of the broadsheets was an article which quoted the MP Nicholas Ridley, a member of Margaret Thatcher's government, as having declared that the government no longer believed my story that I had been tortured. I felt sick: afraid and angry, and perhaps I knew even then that this would destroy my monastic dreams. I made my way to the dining room and as I passed the storeroom I heard the phone ring and went in to answer it. I should explain that the phone was usually answered by the sister who manned the door, but during Mass it was put through to the storeroom. When I picked up the receiver I was surprised to find a member from the Chile Committee for Human Rights asking for me. I experienced immediately the conflict of loyalties which was to plague me for the next few weeks. I knew I should not be taking this call but I hadn't sought it and here I was caught up instantly in the old drama. My friend explained that it was vital that I speak out to defend myself: that silence would be the equivalent of acknowledging the truth of Ridley's allegations. Terrified of being caught in this illicit conversation, I said I had to go and fled to breakfast. No sooner had I begun my cereal, however, than the novice mistress appeared at the dining-room door and beckoned to me imperiously. I followed her, my heart pounding, up to the novitiate where she addressed me, offering me, if I remember her correctly, the option of packing my bags and going then and there or keeping silent and not defending myself. I asked if I could consult Michael Hollings, my priest friend, but was told that I could not. Did I take time to think things through? I don't remember. What I do know is that I chose my monastic vision over my role in the Chile drama and said that I would stay and leave it to her and the prioress. At the time, this seemed the right decision, but it was one that was to make me ill with conflict and worry.

All of that day the press besieged the convent and every few minutes I heard the novice mistress's bell as she was called to the phone yet again. I felt completely desperate, as though I had somehow betrayed all my friends in prison and all political prisoners everywhere. I badly wanted to ask advice of someone wise in both the ways of the spirit and of the world, but this was forbidden to me. I had no real confidence in the convent superiors: I felt they couldn't possibly understand. Years later, my friend Tom said, 'You never really went to Slough, did you?' He meant that I never really trusted myself to the community and I'm sure he was right. Whether I was wrong *not* to trust is another matter and I suspect no one can tell me 'yes' or 'no' over that.

By the following Sunday things had quietened down and I had a reassuring letter from Michael Hollings to say that I was far more powerful in the Chileans' defence staying silent. I suppose because it gave credence to my abdication of human rights lobbying for the monastic life. The Sunday broadsheets, to my great surprise, rose to my defence saying that it was monstrous of the Conservatives to try to rewrite history to suit their own ends and that there was no evidence whatsoever that I was anything but honest. I felt much better when I read these editorials but the damage had been done and about a week later I began to get indigestion. I dosed myself with antacids but it got worse and worse until the very smell of food made me feel ill. By this time it was Lent and it was the community's custom to fast each Friday evening. Somehow, I couldn't cope with the dry bread which was our meal and it would stick in my throat, reminding me of how the dry bread I had in solitary confinement made me gag so that I couldn't swallow it. I must have been pathologically anxious at the time because I would start to panic about supper several hours before. Eventually, I decided that this was ridiculous and went to the novice mistress who, no doubt, saw this as yet another example of my inability to conform. The sister who cooked our supper was therefore instructed to prepare a separate meal for me, which I suppose is what I'd wanted, but the humiliation of it, coupled with the overcooked dry rice and hard-poached egg, nearly choked me anyway!

It wasn't long before I was really unwell with constant severe indigestion and nausea provoked by any food smells. Convinced that I had a duodenal ulcer, I phoned my doctor in Oxford and travelled down to see him. Dr Bent Juel Jensen had known me for twenty years and could see at once that I was in a state. Unable to care for me at a distance he admitted me to one of his beds in the isolation hospital and arranged a barium meal. Sure enough, I had an ulcer, provoked no doubt by the enormous stress of the past few weeks. Not trusting the nuns to look after me, he decided to treat me the old-fashioned way with diet and bed rest, so I spent the next few weeks sleeping, reading and eating frequent bowls of rice pudding, which I adored.

Bent was due to go off on holiday so he left me in the care of his registrar, William, a kindly young man with sophisticated literary tastes who entertained me by reading the poems and plays of T. S. Eliot to me. Perhaps I should explain that the Slade Hospital was a rather leisurely place, a legacy from the days when there were numbers of patients with tuberculosis who spent months or years on bed rest. Now that TB patients could be treated in the community the beds were retained for sporadic cases of infectious disease. I remember William saying that he was going up to the big hospital, the John Radliffe, to hear a lecture about a newly discovered virus called HIV! This was, of course over twenty-five years ago.

One day when William and I were gossiping about things medical, he mentioned the newly developing hospice movement: a radically different way of caring for terminally-ill patients, especially those with cancer. He offered to take me to visit Sir Michael Sobell House, the Oxford NHS hospice, which was situated in the grounds of the Churchill Hospital, my work-place of fifteen years earlier. Thinking that anything would be better than lying in bed, I accepted his offer and that afternoon we set off to visit Dr Robert Twycross, the Medical Director of the hospice.

Twycross was around my age and had been in the medical school a year before me, but I had no memory of him. What I do remember, however, is that as we began our conversation he said, 'I knew you'd come!' I was amazed, for it had never occurred to me to work with the dying: I was far too enthusiastic about saving lives to be interested in those patients who were near to death. When I asked him why, he smiled and said something like, 'With your background it was obvious.' When I think about it now I think he was referring not just to my Chilean experience but to my Christian beliefs, for at that time most of those involved in hospice work were practising, if not ardent, believers. At the time I agreed politely and said I had other plans, never dreaming that Robert and William knew me better than I knew myself.

After three or four weeks' bed rest all my symptoms had gone and I realised that I couldn't stay in the Slade for ever, but dreaded going back to the convent. When my discharge was discussed, therefore, I asked my doctor if he thought it would be a good idea if I had some convalescence before returning to Slough. Bent, now back from his holiday, pronounced this an excellent idea, so when the novice mistress next came to visit me I told her that the doctors thought I should take some convalescence before coming back to the convent. The novice mistress gave a sort of sceptical snort and said mysteriously, 'This raises questions!' Not knowing what she meant, I relaxed thankfully after her departure and had another little nap and another bowl of rice pudding.

Two days later, however, she was back to tell me that she had discussed me with the Reverend Mother and they felt that I was clearly unhappy at Slough and it would be much better if I left.

Now, of course, I can see that they were right, but at the time I was both dismayed and furious. How dare they tell me to leave before my allotted two years were up: how would I finish my novitiate now? And without completing the novitiate successfully, how could I start my own order and become the great monastic foundress which I believed to be my special destiny? Clearly they cared nothing for me and my plans and I felt bitterly rejected. I have only vague memories of the following days and weeks but a kind friend drove me down to Devon to stay with my brother Mike.

I forgot to mention earlier that when I entered the convent in the Autumn of 1978, I had indulged in some dramatic bridge-burning, giving my car away to the impecunious Latin America Centre for Refugees in London and selling my share of the family house to my sister. The proceeds of the sale I used to pay my taxes before giving the rest to those working with Chilean refugees in London. It had all seemed such a good idea at the time, but now I was not only homeless but virtually penniless as well.

A week or so later I had to return to Oxford to have a small gynae operation and, for some reason that I cannot quite remember, arranged to spend the night at Stanbrook Abbey, the Benedictine monastery for women near Worcester. I had stayed at Stanbrook in 1976, the year of my return from Chile, and I think I must have been advised or decided to seek their advice about my monastic future. The advice of Dame Elizabeth Sumner, the Lady Abbess of Stanbrook, is however, graven indelibly upon my memory. Looking down upon me from a great height (she was a very tall woman), she said in her powerful voice, 'What have you been doing?' Miserably I answered that I had been trying to fit myself like a square peg into a round hole. She thought a moment and then gave me the best advice I've ever had: 'Why don't you just be Sheila?'

So that was that: I wasn't meant to be Joan of Arc or St Bernard of Clairvaux, but plain Sheila Cassidy, doctor, writer and broadcaster but most definitely not a nun! After the operation I retired to Devon once more to lick my wounds. My sister-in-law Pat was in Australia for a few weeks so I was able to recuperate slowly in my brother's house. It is hard to convey how traumatic is the re-entry into ordinary life after being confined in a convent. Even after two weeks in Stanbrook in 1961 I almost fell under a car, so unused was I to the pace of 'normal' life. This time I had been 'inside' for eighteen months so my readjustment took time. After a couple of weeks, however, my brother's wife Pat returned and it was time for me to make a move.

Despite the Abbess's wise words I was still reluctant to let go of my monastic dream, so I decided that the obvious thing was to spend a while as a hermit, praying and thinking about my future. With hindsight, I can see that I am no more suited to being a hermit than I was to being a nun, but then, of course, I was blinded by my vision. My brother found me a second-hand caravan and installed me in the field behind his house. By now we were well into spring so caravan dwelling held no fears for me as I began what was to be an exceptionally brief experience as a hermit. Once settled in, I developed my routine: I rose early to pray and recite the morning offices, and then, after breakfast, borrowed my brother's car to drive into the nearest town of Kingsbridge to attend daily Mass. After Mass I would go for a coffee and perhaps visit the Oxfam shop (which, in my celebrity days, I had opened) and buy perhaps a pair of jeans for 50p (after all, I had to support a third-world charity!).

After a few weeks my brother got fed up with being without his car each morning and suggested that perhaps it was time I bought one of my own. (He clearly did not understand that as a hermit I was bound by Holy Poverty and could not possibly *own* a car!) Reluctantly I bought an old van: yet another step back into the real world. After six weeks, not surprisingly, I ran out of money and, after considering what I could do, decided that there was nothing for it but to see if I could get a job in the hospital in Plymouth because I didn't really have enough experience to work as a GP locum. Nervously, for I had been out of medicine for five years and away from British medicine for nine, I phoned Medical Personnel at Freedom Fields Hospital in Plymouth and was told that there was a locum SHO post available in the radiotherapy department the following week. I accepted the job and also a locum in geriatrics to follow on from the first post. I was nervous but thankful: at least I would not have to worry about money for a few weeks. Little did I know, however, that this temporary return to medical practice would lead to so much happiness and more spiritual fulfilment than I could ever have found in the religious life.

21

RETURN TO MEDICINE:
JULY 1980

The first step in my return to the practice of medicine in the UK was an interview with the head of the Plymouth Radiotherapy Department, a delightful, softly spoken doctor called John Brindle. John had been at Oxford several years before me and we had many good friends and memories in common. He seemed pleased to welcome me to his department though he warned me gently that I would be working on equal terms with doctors twenty years my junior and must be careful not to throw my weight about. I assured him that it was years since I had had any authority over anyone and promised that I would be extra careful.

On 1 July 1980 I started as locum SHO on wards 18, 19, 20 at Freedom Fields Hospital in Plymouth and found that it was as if I'd never been away from medicine. I have always loved work on the in-patient wards and was enormously content talking to patients, examining them, writing up their histories, taking their blood and so on. The nurses on the ward were warm and friendly and I got on well with Rob, the other junior doctor. It was not many days before I found myself walking down the hospital corridor whistling cheerfully as I realised that this and not the convent was where I belonged. I wrote piously somewhere that hospital corridors were my cloister and that I 'told' the patients gently and lovingly as a nun 'tells' her beads.

After two weeks in the department I was enjoying myself so much that I persuaded the personnel department to find someone else to do the geriatric locum and let me stay where I was. Not long after that, as I was walking down the corridor, another of the consultants joined me and said something like, 'Dr Cassidy, I like the way you work! Why don't you stay?'

I couldn't have been more surprised, for I had assumed that my somewhat scatty way of working must be irritating all and sundry: but it was not so. I think that what the doctor, Chris Tyrrell, had picked up was the warmth with which I treated the patients, as well as my natural cheerfulness and good humour. To my amazement, he suggested that I should consider radiotherapy as a career and said that I could make the grade as a consultant within four years.

When I had cashed in my superannuation to buy my passage to Chile in 1973, I thought that I was abandoning all chances of a hospital career in the UK, so my whiskers twitched at the suggestion that all was not lost. I should say here that I have always loved hospital life and its people and have never for a minute considered general practice with its endless round of coughs, colds and haemorrhoids. I longed for the drama of acute medicine and surgery and liked nothing better than the excitement of accident and emergency when you never knew from one minute to the next what fate would bring.

Full of enthusiasm at Chris's suggestion I applied for and got the job for which I was doing a locum, so now I was a bona fide member of the department. I lived in the doctors' residence and returned only occasionally to visit my family fifteen miles away.

Having no family in Plymouth and no real home to go to, I spent most of my evenings on the wards, whether I was on call or not. I enjoyed walking slowly round the patients and spent much time talking to those in the side wards, many of whom were terminally ill. Sitting on the side of their beds, with only the bed lamp on, produced a setting of particular intimacy so that the patients often found the courage to ask that most difficult of questions: 'What's going to happen to me?' or 'Am I going to die?'

I should explain that, in the 1980s, it was the norm not to tell patients if they had a fatal illness, lest they 'give up' or, worse still, commit suicide. This was the famous 'conspiracy of silence' in which the patients' doctors and relatives conspired together to 'protect' them from the truth that their disease was incurable. I found this prevarication difficult as I am by nature a very truthful person and when the patients asked me for the truth in this almost confessional setting I felt quite unable to lie. Once I had told a man or woman that their disease could not be cured, I was in quite an awkward situation as I had gone against what my bosses had told them. In order to protect myself I had to enter into a different sort of collusion with the patient who promised not to let on to the boss what he or she knew!

Twenty-five years on, things are very different and it is now the norm to be truthful with patients about their prognosis, though doctors still find it difficult to 'break bad news'. The whole issue of doctors' and nurses' communication with their patients remains a major subject for teaching and research and I have been involved in the former for many years.

Once I was established in my post, Dr Brindle arranged for me to have tutoring to prepare me for the preliminary exams of the Royal College of Radiologists and Oncologists. In order to understand radiotherapy I had to learn basic physics and I found myself too tired to study and quite unable to retain the facts from one tutorial to another. I persevered, however, for I was finding working with cancer patients increasingly interesting and rewarding and liked the idea of a career in oncology.

After a year of living in one hospital room, I decided it was time I found myself somewhere to live and set out to find a flat to rent. Still determined to be holier than anyone else, I made a decision never to own property again. When I was complaining about the difficulty of finding a place to rent, my junior doctor colleague asked me, 'Why don't you get a mortgage?' I realised that I might just as well do what my fellow doctors did and approached a couple of estate agents for a flat to buy. My first intention was to live in a poor area: after all, if my nun friends chose to live alongside the poor and the oppressed in Chile or the ghettos of New York, surely I should too. The nurses, however, were scornful of my intentions and said I would live in constant fear of being mugged or robbed.

My fate was decided, however, on the day the estate agent rang me and said, in a delighted voice, 'Dr Cassidy, we've found *your* flat!' I asked her what she meant but she insisted that I go for a viewing. So that afternoon, my fellow SHO Rob Kneen and I climbed the seventy-two steps to inspect an attic flat overlooking Plymouth's magnificent harbour. I could not believe my luck, for here was a two-bedroom flat with a panoramic view of the harbour and the ocean beyond, all for the price of seventeen thousand pounds. Rob and I fell about laughing with delight and I told the agent that she was right: this was indeed *my* flat.

Some time in 1981 I set up house, furnishing the flat with a motley collection of family and second-hand furniture. It was in fact extremely difficult to get any furniture at all up the narrow servants' staircase and my dining-room table nearly got stuck halfway up. Once installed, I was blissfully happy, for there is nothing I like better than 'playing houses'. Sometimes I think that I should have been an interior decorator, for I love choosing furniture, colours and fabrics.

At this point in my life, however, my desires were reined in by my notion of gospel living, inherited mainly from my monk friend Tom Cullinan. In an effort to keep up with him I made the decision to have no vacuum cleaner, no washing machine and no television. I laid no carpets on the stairs and swept the bare boards with a brush, choking the while on the dust. What really defeated me, however, was the washing, for I couldn't seem to get anything clean. After a couple of months I acquired a cleaner (giving much-needed employment to the poor!) and asked her if she would wash my sheets, towels and shirts. This she did willingly but the cost seemed to mount up and one day I went out and bought a half-size automatic washing machine instead. I never looked back and the machine worked perfectly for twenty years without a single service.

The ultimate collapse of my ascetic resolve came when Evelyn Waugh's classic *Brideshead Revisited* was serialised for television, and without further ado I rushed out and bought a TV. Now, twenty and more years later I am a total addict and spend my evenings glued to medical and police soaps like *Casualty* and *The Bill*. At least in this I am in solidarity with the unemployed and the poor! Somewhere along the line I acquired carpet on the stairs and a vacuum cleaner to keep them looking good. The real fun, however, came when I started to take down the ceilings and move the walls about. More of that later.

Sometime during 1980 I made a new friend, a very clever and creative woman called Phoebe-Ann Caldwell. Phoebe-Ann had lost her husband a few months earlier and was glad of a friend with whom to play houses, go walking and shop. She was part of the healthcare world, working as a therapist with adults with profound learning difficulties in the Bristol region. She came to Plymouth on my weekends off and we took picnics on the moors and explored the local beauty spots. Phoebe-Ann was a great lover of the Yorkshire Dales and we had many happy holidays in Littondale, exploring all the local markets and tourist shops.

I remember one holiday during which I had to prepare for a retreat to be given at the Corrymeela Centre for reconciliation in Ballycastle, Northern Ireland. For days I struggled with my Bible but could find no appropriate theme save that of light. Then, fossicking about in the gift shops of Skipton I came across some enchanting rainbow candles. All at once I knew that I had my theme: rainbows, the sign of God's covenant with his people. I bought all the candles they had – about fifty – and carried them off to our rented cottage where I searched my concordance for biblical references to rainbows. To my surprise there are only four references: the rainbow in the sky after the flood; Ezekiel's theophany by the river Chebar; a brief reference in Ecclesiastes; and the glimpse of heaven afforded to St John on the island of Patmos. From these small fish of inspiration I elaborated my 'Theology of Rainbows' which was warmly welcomed at Corrymeela and came in useful for various other sermons and talks. (The theology of rainbows, as I mentioned earlier, weaves together the fact that we are called by name (like Ezekiel), into the unknown (like Abraham), with no promise from God save that he will be with us, whatever happens.)

Phoebe-Ann has moved on to great things in her work with the handicapped and is much sought after for her knowledge and expertise by those in this field. She now lives in her beloved North, in Lancashire, so our paths rarely cross, but we have made a promise to meet up this year.

Towards the end of 1981 I learned that Plymouth was soon to have its own hospice. I was not particularly interested because I still had my sights set upon being an oncologist. One day, however, I received a phone call inviting me to become the medical director of the new St Luke's Hospice when it opened the following January. I was amazed, for I had never before been 'head hunted' for anything. At first, I thought I would get my oncology exams and then move into hospice work but I soon realised that if I refused this job they would surely give it to someone else and, in four years' time, there would be no place for me. The other determining factor was that I was making heavy weather of the physics and it was by no means certain that I had what it took to pass the exams. In my family the women have a taste for books and poetry while the men have a flair for maths. I, alas, was virtually innumerate and I decided that I'd better accept the hospice offer for there would probably never be a better one.

After eighteen months as SHO in oncology, I left the hospital and the security of the NHS to work for a charity, with all the politics that that involved. I was to spend eleven years as Medical Director of St Luke's until the very people who had given me the job decided that they would prefer someone else and I returned to spend the rest of my career in the Plymouth oncology unit.

22

❧ ⚬ ❧

ST LUKE'S HOSPICE –
THE BEGINNING:
1982

The British hospice movement was well underway when we opened St Luke's in Plymouth in February 1982. The first UK hospice was The Hostel of God, now Trinity Hospice, Clapham, which opened in 1891; it was followed by St Luke's Home for the Dying Poor in West London in 1893. St Joseph's Hospice in Hackney opened in 1905, but it wasn't until the 1960s that Dr Cicely Saunders, pioneer of today's hospice movement, opened St Christopher's Hospice at Sydenham, after learning how to care for the dying from the nuns at St Luke's Home. By the 1980s there were hospices in all the major British cities and the basic methods of pain and symptom control were well established.

In order to prepare myself for my new job I spent a rather lonely two weeks as locum medical director at the Mount Edgcumb Hospice in St Austell in Cornwall and then did a brief tour of a few of the better-known units in the UK. This latter trip was time well spent, for I had the opportunity to meet a number of the key people in the movement: Derek Doyle in Edinburgh, Robert Twycross in Oxford and Eric Wilkes in Sheffield. Most of these hospice founders were highly charismatic people and many were driven by their Christian faith to care for the dying. It is worth noting at this point that hospices are started by men and women with the enthusiasm, drive and vision to create something out of nothing, but these people do not always have the tact and other diplomatic qualities required to run an organisation in the long term. Pioneers are not necessarily good maintainers.

On my return to Plymouth I found that the matron initially appointed by the Hospice Council of Management was now considered to be unsatisfactory and a new one was to be appointed. I persuaded one of my favourite nurses in the oncology unit to apply but, arriving for interview with her hair loose to her waist, she stood no chance against the Council's favoured candidate, Valerie Oliver, an experienced community nurse of mature years and impeccable grooming. During the years that followed, I found it increasingly difficult to work with Valerie because of personality differences but there is no doubt that she established a high standard of nursing and patient care right from the first day. When the different nurses had been appointed, the beds made and the cupboards stocked, we were ready to receive our first patient, a farmer's wife with a terrible ulcerated malignancy of the vulva. 'Elizabeth' was an ideal candidate for hospice care, requiring good pain control and highly skilled nursing. After her came two other patients and then some more, and we were really up and running.

During those first few months we ran seven beds, which were increased to ten in the Autumn as demand grew. The hospice was a converted family house, which gave it a nice homely feel but made it difficult to run as a nursing home. Space was at a premium: there were two three-bedded rooms and one single upstairs, and one three-bedded room downstairs. The office was tiny and contained the locked drug cupboard, the drugs trolley and a desk for one, so we used the next-door bathroom for meetings and as an overflow office.

With hindsight, it's amazing that we performed as well as we did. None of us had done hospice work before and several of the senior nurses had only recently returned to work after rearing their children. If I didn't know what to do for a patient I rang up other hospice people around the country and made notes of their advice. I read Cicely Saunders' and Twycross's books as if they were the Bible and went to any conference that was available. I was the only doctor and was employed for five, three-and-a-half-hour 'sessions' – around twenty hours a week, although I once calculated that I worked ninety.

The local general practitioners were very generous and volunteered to be on call for the hospice at night and at the weekends without charge, but if there were any major difficulties the nurses usually phoned me. On Mondays and Tuesdays I worked at the hospice in the morning, the hospital in the afternoon, then returned to the hospice in the evening to admit any new patients and sort out problems. I really enjoyed the work but the responsibility of being the only doctor lay heavily upon my shoulders and I became increasingly stressed. Added to my clinical load was an increasing burden teaching about hospice work. Many of the para-medical practitioners such as physiotherapists, social workers and speech therapists were interested in learning about the new specialty and I soon had a sizeable teaching commitment in Plymouth, Devon and Cornwall. Added to this was the human rights lecturing and religious broadcasting, which of course I did in my own time. I was very happy to give these talks but found myself getting increasingly anxious before lecturing. Once again I found that I had trouble sleeping and became caught up in a vicious circle of being too anxious to sleep and too tired to perform well the following day. It didn't help that I was increasingly at odds with Valerie, the matron, and used to let off steam talking about my difficulties with a couple of the senior nurses. There were also minor difficulties between other members of staff and I realised that the stress of working full time with such desperately ill people probably manifested itself as conflict between carers. Some years later I read papers and a book by Toronto nurse-psychologist Mary Vachon, who had become an expert in understanding occupational stress in such emotionally highly charged units as hospices and intensive care units. In all these situations the practitioners would insist, 'It's not the patients that stress me, it's my colleagues, it's the system.'

Accepting that stress was endemic in the profession was not the same as curing it. There was much talk in the 1980s about support groups but we never really found them helpful. Nurses on duty declared themselves too busy to attend, while those off duty were, not unreasonably, unwilling to come in on their day off. When people *did* come to the group it was usually a mixture of junior and senior nurses and none of us could really declare that we were irritated to screaming point by A or B or C, particularly if that person was a senior member of staff. The Methodist minister who was facilitating the group did his best with us but eventually the group died a natural death. Things were better for everyone, however, a couple of years later when I found a therapist away from the hospice to whom I could unload, so my temptation to gossip with the senior nurses was reduced.

My stress and overwork led to a head-on collision with my bosses one evening at one of the meetings of the hospice Council. It was August and a week or so previously I had gone to visit a cancer patient at the nearby Freedom Fields Hospital. After I had talked to the man he asked me if I would see another patient with whom he had become friendly. Professional etiquette, of course, forbade me from accepting a referral from a patient, but I was intrigued and it seemed churlish to refuse. The man, whom I shall call Peter, as I have long since forgotten his name, turned out to be an Anglo-Chilean businessman in his forties who had been taken ill while visiting the UK. He was suffering from malignant hypertension (very high blood pressure) which had caused him to become suddenly blind. Medically, he was stable on medication, but socially he was in dire straits as he had had no input from the services for the blind and his return ticket to Chile was due to expire in less than two weeks. I spoke to the nurses but was told that his consultant was on holiday and that there were no plans to get him mobile or reading Braille. Because he was both English and Chilean, I not only empathised with Peter but felt moved to help him. So, without further thought, I offered to admit him to the hospice for rehabilitation. The nurses were delighted and Peter was shipped over to the hospice before the day was out.

As luck would have it, we had just the accommodation that Peter needed because the ground-floor sitting room at the hospice was in the process of being converted into a ward but was not yet ready for occupation. There was, however, a bed and a chair, which was all Peter needed. The first thing we did was to buy him a tape recorder and help him make an audio tape to send to his wife, a Chilean, explaining what had happened, for he had not been able to telephone her. The following morning, I made contact with the services for the blind and persuaded them that Peter needed to be seen that day, as there was unlikely to be any help when he returned to Chile. That afternoon, I met Peter and his therapist in the street as she taught him to walk with his white stick. Within days he had been introduced to Braille and taught to use his tape recorder on his own. It remained only for us to obtain a three months' supply of his anti-hypertensive medication and he was ready to return home. I can't recall exactly how I got the pills: probably by leaning on both the hospital pharmacist and Terry, our own warm-hearted local chemist.

The nurses and I were extremely pleased with ourselves about the whole affair but I had not reckoned with the ire of the Council when they found out what I had done. I can't remember if I included Peter's story in my monthly report or whether someone had reported me but I was severely admonished for admitting a non-cancer patient on the grounds that I was contravening the rules of the hospice and betraying our supporters. (The real reason for the Chairman's anxiety, I think, was that he thought I had harboured a Chilean terrorist.) If I'd been strong and a man I'd probably have told the Chairman that I was Medical Director and it was my decision which patients to admit, but I was neither, so I burst into floods of tears and flounced out. No one followed to comfort or reason with me but they did eventually agree to pay another doctor for an extra seven hours of medical time per week so that I did not have to come back to the hospice in the evening after I had done my hospital outpatient work.

One of my problems with the Council was that, although I loved the clinical work at the hospice and was good at it, I had little interest in the administration and even less in fundraising. I was never really at ease with the members of the Council because most of them were business-men with whom I had very little in common. For many years I also had a problem with those whom I perceived as authority figures, which included consultants, bank managers, solicitors, headmasters and the like. Not only was I afraid of them but I secretly despised them for power dressing in their pinstriped suits and smart ties. I also loathed business meetings and failed to attend if I could find an excuse not to. As I said before, those who have the energy to get a venture off the ground are not necessarily the right people to run it long term!

It was round about this time in 1983 that I became friendly with Father Ronnie McAinsh, novice master at the local Redemptionist monastery. Ronnie is a Scotsman and a trained psychotherapist and I sought his help as a spiritual director. One day when I was particularly fraught he told me that I should make a retreat and arranged for me to see a Father Michael Ivens SJ, who was based at St Beuno's, a Jesuit retreat centre near St Asaph in North Wales.

St Beuno's is a massive Victorian pile built to house the dozens of young men who entered the Society of Jesus in the 1900s. When these 'vocations' dried up in the 1950s it was converted to become a retreat house, which it remains to this day. The house is situated on a hillside overlooking the ravishingly beautiful Clwyd Valley and it is a marvellous place to make a retreat. I was struck at once by the generous proportions of the building: big rooms and wide sunny corridors arranged around a central quadrangle. The chapel too was spacious and I felt instantly at home in a monastic (as opposed to a domestic) kind of way.

Father Michael Ivens was a delight: a quietly spoken, slightly dishevel-led man in a woolly jumper and sandals with socks. He was welcoming without being effusive and I warmed to him straight away. I had yet to learn that Michael was famous in Jesuit circles for his intellect and wit and was regarded as being one of the wisest and most intuitive of spiritual directors in the Society of Jesus (the Jesuits). Michael visited me twice each day and I talked about my medical work and the lecturing, the TV programmes I recorded, the insomnia and the tension at the hospice, and so on. I spent a happy day constructing a massive chart of all my engagements, colour coded as medical, religious, apostolic. I can remember Michael's gentle irony as he commented, 'It seems to me that you are living at least three lives at once,' but even then I did not get the message that I was doing too much.

Jesuits are well used to idealistic, neurotic, over-worked men and women, and eventually, when I had talked myself dry, Michael persuaded me to spend the last few days of my time there in complete silence.

I don't recall now what emerged from this particular retreat except the always broken resolution to do less lecturing and spend more time in prayer. I went to St Beuno's regularly after this initial visit and Michael became a much-loved mentor to me. He often gave me the task of retracing my own 'salvation history': the movement of the Holy Spirit in the various twists and turns of my life. This exercise always led me to a deep feeling of gratitude to God and ultimately to a sense of peace.

Ignatian spirituality is, at first sight, very different from Benedictine but I found myself deeply at home in both. The Jesuits speak of 'finding God in all things' and of living a life of action in the world, sustained by contemplation, while the Benedictines live somewhat apart from the world, offering their prayer and their work to God. One of my monastic friends used to talk to me of the desert and the marketplace: when one is in the desert, in solitude, on retreat, he said, one worries that one should be out in the marketplace, tending the sick, feeding the hungry, teaching the unlettered and so on; but then, when one pitches one's tent in the city, the desert calls with its silence and emptiness so redolent of the Divine.

I love 'the desert' of being on retreat and used to lie on the floor in the dark in the little individual prayer chapels at St Beuno's and know that prostration was the only attitude to adopt before the Throne. The mistake I made in entering the convent was that I thought I could live this life full time: but I can't. I hunger for solitude and silence but if I have it for too long I become inward looking and soul-scratching, anxiously picking at my wounds and worrying about my soul. My primary call is clearly to the 'marketplace' and I am born to wash feet and tend the lepers' wounds. St Paul was so right when he talked about there being many gifts but the same Spirit.

The problem of the Ignatian way, of course, is how to keep the contemplation going in the midst of action and I have struggled with this all my life. From time to time I would establish a routine of daily prayer – sometimes as much as an hour a day – but no sooner had I congratulated myself on being a contemplative in the world than the whole thing would fall apart and I would feel bad again. The best way for me during these busy professional years was to pray when I was able and take myself off on retreat every three or four months. My theory was that if I went up the mountain to seek the Lord, that is, if I carved precious time for God out of my busy life, he would come halfway down to meet me. I still believe that, because I have never yet been disappointed.

In 1984, two years after we had opened the hospice, I was invited to lecture about my Chile experience in Toronto and took the time out as annual leave to go. When I returned, however, I was summoned to talk to the two medical members of the hospice Council who told me that my post was to be upgraded from clinical assistant to consultant and I would be expected to work full time at the hospice. I was told that if I accepted I would have the same study leave allowance as hospital consultants and that leave to undertake academic engagements (in my case lecturing) away from Plymouth would be negotiable between me and the hospice.

With hindsight, it was a generous offer but I was angry with them because I saw it as a deliberate move to clip my wings. Although I worked far more than the eight or nine sessions for which I was now employed, I was able to take time out when I needed to and, in particular, I took a day off each week which felt, at the time, to be vital to my survival. I explained that I preferred to work part time but the two men were adamant: it was a take-it-or-leave-it offer. Either I went full time or I left. Feeling both trapped and abused I agreed to their proposal and knuckled down to working full time.

Although I think the Council was pleased with the idea that it had more control over me, nothing really changed except that I was paid a substantially higher salary. Three weeks' study leave a year was more than I had taken previously and I still had the freedom, within my contract, to lecture both at home and abroad. This issue of my lecturing absences remained a difficult one for the next eight years: I know that people muttered about it behind my back but no one ever challenged me to my face or asked me to stay at home more.

Although I knew I was an excellent lecturer, I continued to suffer severe performance anxiety and nearly always slept very badly before an important engagement. The difficulty of this was heightened by the fact that I was often a guest in people's homes and I worried terribly about waking them or their dogs. As my fear of making a fool of myself heightened, I became an increasingly neurotic traveller, refusing duvets because I was too hot, dragging my mattress onto the floor if the bed sagged, and carrying with me supplies of cake, muesli, hot chocolate and whisky to sustain myself during the long hours of the night. When I contrast the emotional freedom with which I now travel and my ability to sleep almost anywhere at any time, I realise how unwell I was.

Absurdly, though I sought help from my GP frequently, no one diagnosed that I was depressed or considered that I might be suffering from post-traumatic stress. My doctor willingly gave me sleeping pills: at first temazepam and then, as I became more desperate, the 'date-rape' drug flunitrazepam (Rohypnol). Both of these drugs worked well at first but within a few days I became tolerant of them and slept as badly as ever.

When I talked about my difficulty with friends they were sympathetic but helpless. Some made me furious by suggesting that perhaps I didn't need to sleep and should use the night to write my books. Even I didn't realise that I was depressed, attributing my low mood and despair to lack of sleep.

One Saturday morning in December 1984, however, my luck changed and I met the first man who understood how desperately I needed help. His name was James Thompson and he was lecturing on the threat of nuclear war; something he said about anxiety caught my interest and, in the lunch break, I joined the small group around him. He was talking about his work with victims of torture and, my ears flapping, I asked him as casually as I could whether he was working with any of the Chilean refugees. His gaze immediately focused on me and he said bluntly, 'Who are you?' I told him my name and realised that he knew of my Chilean connection. There came then a brief moment when we were alone and he said, I think, 'Have you talked about it in therapy?' I said 'No', to which he replied firmly 'You should!' I responded 'Why?' and he replied with an answer which I have never forgotten: 'It's cheaper than keeping it under wraps!'

In January of 1985 I went to London to see James Thompson at the Middlesex Hospital and I still recall my embarrassment and indignation when the receptionist asked me if I was a patient. I admitted crossly that I was but made sure she knew I was a doctor and therefore a person of some importance! James is a clinical psychologist and psychotherapist who is part of an increasingly large network of therapists dedicated to the treatment of men and women who have encountered severe psychic trauma. Examples of this are the survivors of the football stadium disaster at Hillsborough, the sinking of the ferry, the *Herald of Free Enterprise*, the Kings Cross fire and so on. In 2005, as I write, the management of post-traumatic stress disorder (PTSD) is of intense worldwide interest, especially after the attacks of 9/11 and 7 July, but in the mid-1980s the problem was less well known and I was enormously lucky to be seen by James.

On that first visit, he asked me to tell him my story, from childhood to that day and sat patiently for nearly four hours as I struggled to articulate the difficulties of my childhood, my love of Consuelo, the dramas of prison and my current difficulties at the hospice. When at last I had finished he was grey with fatigue, and I realise now that he was probably more affected by listening to my story than I had been in the telling of it. The truth was that I had told my story in public so often that I had unconsciously dissociated the narration of my experience from the memory of how I felt at the time. The terrible fear that I had felt in Chile was locked away deep in my psyche and emerged only occasionally when something triggered it. One such event occurred as I was driving to work: I passed a woman with a child in a pushchair and, as I drew level with her, her petticoat fell to the ground, the elastic having presumably given way. As I watched in mild amusement I was conscious of a voice in my head saying in Spanish, '*Saccarse la ropa*', 'Take off your clothes', and I was instantly back with my torturers in the Villa Grimaldi, quite powerless and sick with terror. Years later when I tried to deliberately access the memories of torture with my psychiatrist I became familiar with the feelings of nausea which accompanied recovery of the fear. More of that later.

I saw James a few more times but the distance between London and Plymouth made regular therapy impracticable. He arranged, therefore, that I should see a friend and colleague of his, Jim Drewery, who was head of the clinical psychology unit in Exeter, only forty minutes' drive from Plymouth. In his letter of referral he described me as having an 'agitated depression', and, absurdly, I felt deeply ashamed. Little did I know at the time that I was embarking upon a journey which would lead to my becoming a psychotherapist myself.

In 1984 I began to have weekly therapy with Jim, a gentle Scotsman whom I came to know and love as a friend. Only my secretary knew what the initials signified in my diary and she covered for me each week if anyone asked where I was. With Jim I talked about my life, past and present, and he helped me to understand that the way I was currently living was profoundly unhealthy. I will never forget the day he turned on me in exasperation and said, 'Can't you see that you are destroying yourself!'

Jim was deeply concerned at my levels of stress and told me in no uncertain terms that I must give up lecturing about my experiences in Chile. He likened my forays into the human rights world to the missions of the bomber pilots during the Second World War: the fear involved in each raid accumulated until they could no longer cope and had to be taken off active duty. I found his suggestion very difficult to accept because to refuse to involve myself in this work felt like a betrayal, not only of the Chilean people in particular, but of all persecuted people in general.

Each week as our session ended, Jim would ask me what I had planned for the weekend and little by little I learned that human rights lecturing incurred his disapproval while plans for fun and recreation elicited a 'Good! Excellent!' I learned, too, that it was good to treat myself and started to spend more money on food and clothes.

At first, Jim's ideas seemed in direct opposition to my religious beliefs. I was, I think, convinced that I was called by God to work harder, pray longer and generally be holier than anyone else! There is a famous prayer attributed to St Ignatius of Loyola, the founder of the Jesuits, which goes something like this:

Lord Jesus, teach me to be generous:

To give and not to count the cost,
to fight and not to heed the wounds,
to work and not to seek for rest,
to seek only to do thy holy will.

I used to think that this was a wonderful prayer but, alas, I now see that it is crazy, for it fails to take into account our human need for rest, for time out and for fun. I was, without realising it, absurdly deluded, believing at some unconscious level that I could save the oppressed people of Chile and the dying of Plymouth almost single handed! I should have remembered the wisdom of Dame Elizabeth, Abbess of Stanbrook, when she said to me, 'Why don't you just be Sheila?'

The trouble was, that was who I *was* in the late 1980s and early 90s. I was Medical Director of St Luke's Hospice in Plymouth, but that was only my 'day job'. Although I eventually stopped lecturing about Chile I soon became a regular national lecturer on emotional distress in the dying, an occasional preacher on prayer and suffering and also a religious broadcaster. My diaries from that period are a jumbled mass of engage-ments, medical and non-medical, religious and secular, and I wonder now not only how I survived but how on earth I got away with it for so many years.

23

ST LUKE'S EXPANDS:
1985

Meanwhile, the work of the hospice went from strength to strength. At the beginning there had been two community nurses, funded by Cancer Relief Macmillan, Jenny Herbert and Lucy Hulbert, who worked in the community, liaising with the general practitioners and visiting the terminally ill in their own homes. In those early days I met with the two of them each week and we talked through their case load and any difficulties they were encountering with colleagues. It was a rich time of sharing and I greatly enjoyed it. As the work increased, more Macmillan nurses were appointed and they formed a team on their own. Those of us who worked in the inpatient unit also met weekly for a 'case conference' to discuss the current patients and any who had died recently and, when time permitted, I taught all the nurses, helping them to understand why the patients had the symptoms that they did.

My assistant doctors came and went, although two of them became permanent members of the hospice staff. The first of these was Dr Michael Fell, a tall thin man who had retired from being a country GP. We all adored Michael and marvelled at the love with which he treated the patients. He was, I think, a real saint, incredibly self-effacing and humble yet ready to stand his ground if he believed something was wrong.

The other doctor was a woman, Dr Mary Burnell Nugent, a bright young married GP who also came to be passionate about care of the dying and who eventually made palliative care her career, succeeding me when I left the hospice.

As our expertise increased, we were referred more and more patients until it became clear that we must expand as soon as possible. John Gorton, our larger-than-life administrator, launched a fundraising appeal and we made plans to move. At first we looked for a large building but then the Council decided that we should purpose-build and persuaded the City Fathers to give us a piece of land overlooking the sea: the new St Luke's was to be built on a high promontory with stunning views over the harbour and beyond.

By 1987, the new hospice was complete: a long two-storey building with twenty beds, a lecture room and all the offices we thought we need-ed at the time. We were enormously excited at the idea of moving and I wanted to make high theatre of it with an elephant and clowns. When the day came, however, it was a question of a fleet of ambulances and lorries, with the rest of us following on in our cars.

A few weeks before the move we took on our first doctor apprentice in the form of Dr Marie Frings, a delightful Belgian woman in her thirties. Marie was interested in palliative care and had been advised to visit me because she, like me, was particularly interested in spiritual issues. When she wrote to me I responded warmly and invited her to stay the night – but, as the date drew near, I panicked about entertaining her. This pattern of behaviour was a familiar one: assuming it would be discourteous to ask visitors to find their own accommodation, I offered a hospitality which I later regretted.

On the day that Dr Frings was due to arrive I reread her letter and decided that she was probably in her late fifties and incredibly worthy and I would be stuck with her all that evening and the following day as well. It was, however, too late to retract my offer, so I went shopping to cheer myself up. By happy coincidence, she arrived outside my door just as I was unloading a collection of bedding plants from the local garden centre so I was able to enlist her help in carrying them up the seventy-two steps to my flat. Luckily for me, Marie was only in her thirties and extremely strong and willing, so I forgot about being anxious as we planted up my roof garden together. The following day I showed her round the hospice and answered as many of her questions as I could before she left for Newcastle to visit the hospice there. A month or so later Marie returned to Plymouth to spend the next six months with us at St Luke's. A natural with the patients, she fitted in well with the staff and went on to start a hospice herself in Charleroi in Belgium and another in the town of Soigny.

Moving to a new and purpose-built hospice was exciting but the real task to be achieved was the integration of a large number of new staff to service the increase in beds. All went smoothly enough but there was no denying that the 'new hospice' was very different from the old. Jim Copper, a consultant in healthcare of the elderly who worked some week-ends for us as a volunteer doctor, summed up the change in atmosphere when he said, 'I do hope the hospice doesn't lose its air of happy chaos.' The nurses who had been with St Luke's since it started would mutter sadly that things were not the same, that the hospice had lost some of its warmth and informality. True as that may be, the really important fact was that we could now treat twice the number of patients in greatly improved facilities, so I for one had no regrets.

The new St Luke's was a state-of-the-art hospice. There were twice the number of beds as in the old hospice and the staff numbers were increased accordingly. A number of new nurses were employed but I was able to keep the same medical team by increasing the hours of my two assistants Michael and Mary. Although I did not realise it, this step was to radically alter the dynamics of the medical team and, eventually, bring about my own downfall.

When I began as Medical Director of St Luke's in 1982 I was the only doctor and the nurses gladly fitted in with my somewhat erratic hours. In particular, they liked to give the patients the opportunity to sleep on, if they could, in the mornings, which suited me as I too liked a leisurely start to the day. By 10.30 the patients had been washed and fed and made comfortable and I discussed their progress with the nurse in charge over a cup of coffee. After that we 'played doctors and nurses', visiting each patient in turn, examining them if necessary and reviewing their treat-ment. This too was a leisurely process and I developed the ability to change like a chameleon, teasing some patients, playing with the cat on another's bed, or sitting quietly with those who needed to weep.

It was very different from hospital medicine but just as serious. Our aim, as Cicely Saunders once put it, was to help people to *live* until they died. This required skilled symptom control, meticulous nursing and careful psycho-social management. It did not take me long to learn that you cannot practise good hospice medicine without understanding what cancer does to the human body, and I taught my assistants and the nurses to question the mechanism of each symptom so that we might better understand how to treat it.

When Ann, my first assistant, was appointed in 1982, she came only three afternoons a week, so I remained very much in charge. Later, Mary and Michael also worked part time so no one questioned my authority. When we moved to the new hospice, however, Mary and Michael, each having doubled their hours, wanted to establish a more regular pattern of working: in particular, they wanted to start the day earlier. At the old hospice, they had always worked in the afternoons, so my arriving late in the morning had never been an issue. Now, however, they insisted that we should discuss the patients at the start of the day's work and I grudgingly agreed to be in by 9.30.

If this sounds late by hospital standards, of course it is, but by now I was suffering from severe chronic insomnia and found it increasingly difficult to pull myself together in the mornings. The result was that, however hard I tried, I was nearly always five or ten minutes late, something which irritated my colleagues on a daily basis. The other issue was one which I remained blind to for years: before I went to the ward meeting I always picked up my post and whenever there was a break in the meeting (e.g. a phone call) I would open and read the most interesting looking of the letters.

As the years passed and hospice education flourished I received an increasing number of invitations to lecture at home and abroad. Had I had any sense, I would have kept these strictly to myself, but I was naive in the ways of team dynamics and would exclaim with delight: 'Guess what! I've got an invitation to lecture in Australia!' With hindsight I can see how these extra-mural activities irritated my colleagues: not only was I not there in the hospice doing the work I was paid for, but I was travelling to exotic places, having fun and, they assumed, being paid richly for the privilege, while they were slaving away, keeping the home fires burning. Although in the eleven years that I was Medical Director, no member of the staff or Council questioned my absences or said that I was taking too much leave, I picked up on the general feeling that some people were not content with my performance. This produced in me the feeling that both Valerie and the Council were against me and I began to feel increasingly threatened. I suppose, if I'd had any sense, I'd have cut down my lecturing but the letters were so persuasive and the lure of foreign travel almost impossible to resist.

I see now that the formalising of the hospice was my personal undoing. Caring for more patients demanded greater efficiency of both nurses and medical staff. A good doctor and an inspiring lecturer I might be, but that was no longer enough, for I still had no real interest in management and was irritating my medical colleagues by frequent absences to lecture. What no one at the hospice knew, for I dared not tell, was that I was becoming increasingly anxious and depressed and had frequent suicidal thoughts. The more I lectured, the less I slept and the more desperate I became, but I still had a deep instinct to keep my difficulties to myself for I believed that the Council would be happy to see me go. I remember seeing a poster in another hospice director's office: it read, 'Just because I'm paranoid, it doesn't mean they are not out to get me!'

As my depression worsened, I'd sit at the open window of my attic flat and think about throwing myself out, or I'd go out to walk by the sea at dawn and think, 'If I swam out and out and out, I'd drown.' One weekend I drove to St Beuno's and everything I saw made me think of suicide: a rope from a skylight suggested hanging, while the red letters saying POISON on the lavatory cleaner suggested a toxic death.

If this was post-traumatic stress, I had only a few of the signs: agitation and insomnia, but no flashbacks and no torture-related nightmares. Some years before, my hospital boss had arranged for me to see a local psychiatrist who, when I told him all I was doing, asked me coldly (or so it felt to me) why I did it. At first I was struck dumb: how could he not understand that I was Chile's Joan of Arc and Devon's Cicely Saunders, driven like the prophet to proclaim good news to the poor and freedom to captives? At the time I found him unhelpful, though we later worked together and become good friends, when, perhaps, I was more open to the possibility that I was my own worst enemy.

Sometime in 1989, my friend and spiritual mentor Michael Ivens became ill with a tumour of the pituitary gland, which at first seriously impaired his eyesight. Although the surgeons were able to remove most of it, the damage incurred meant that he was no longer able to cope with the stress of retreat-giving and was forced into an early retirement. This meant that he could no longer act as my mentor and he suggested I contact his great friend and collaborator Father Gerard Hughes sj.

Gerry lived with the Jesuit community at Manresa House in Harborne, on the outskirts of Birmingham. It was, of course, a far cry from the rural beauty of the Clwyd Valley but I soon came to feel at home there and there was a big park nearby where I could walk and contemplate the ducks on their pond. I came to love the Jesuit way of giving retreatants a couple of excerpts from the Scriptures to prompt their reflections and occasionally I drew the gospel scenes, which made them much more vivid.

More than the gospels, however, I loved the prophets, especially Isaiah with whom I had become familiar in the convent. One day, when we were thinking about 'call' (as in vocation) Gerry gave me Isaiah 6 to read. This is the marvellous passage in which Isaiah encounters God in the Temple. It is one of those spectacular theophanies in which the Lord is surrounded by angels and the Temple is filled with smoke. Isaiah is overcome by awe and declares his unworthiness in the presence of the Divine:

> 'What a wretched state I am in! I am lost,
> for I am a man of unclean lips
> and I live among a people of unclean lips,
> and my eyes have looked at the King, Yahweh Saboath.'
>
> (Isaiah 6:5)

The Lord responds to Isaiah by sending a seraph with a burning coal to cleanse his lips and then declares, 'Your sin is taken away.' Before Isaiah has time to reflect upon his changed state, a challenge is issued: 'I heard the voice of the LORD saying: "Whom shall I send? Who will be our messenger?"' (Isaiah 6:8).

This passage always sends shivers down my spine for I spent so many years of my life struggling with what I saw to be my own call to religious life. Isaiah's reply is like Mary's 'Fiat' (Latin for 'acceptance') at the annunciation. He answers: 'Here I am, LORD. Send me.' I find these words incredibly moving and I spent much of that day thinking about it. It was during that night, however, that I had a leap of understanding that has stayed with me to this day. I woke from sleep and, rather to my irritation, felt obliged to spend some time in prayer. Sighing, I hauled myself out of bed and, lighting a candle, settled down to pray. It was then, I think, that I was given, or anyway thought of, the image of the 'wheelchair God' that I mentioned earlier. The next day, I drew it and the significance became clearer.

I drew a vague figure in a wheelchair sitting sadly at the bottom of some steps leading up to a house in which there was a party going on. The person in the wheelchair could not leave it and climb the steps to join the people in the house, so he had to send a messenger. I saw the amazing paradox of the all-powerful God unable to come personally to heal the sick, forgive sinners and comfort the afflicted as Jesus had done in Galilee because he is no longer of this world. We, therefore, are his messengers: the emissaries of our wheelchair God, sent in spite of our unclean lips into the schools, hospitals and prisons of the world. At last I understood that to restrict the meaning of 'vocation' to religious life was nonsense. Like the prophets, like people of all time, we are called to use our gifts wherever they are most needed.

If ever I am tempted to regret my long neurotic journey into and then out of the convent I remember two things: I would never have learned that I didn't belong there if I hadn't tried the life and, more important, nowhere else would I have received such an amazing exposure to the Christian Scriptures old and new. The latter has provided the inspiration upon which I have drawn for my preaching, broadcasting, writing and spiritual care over the past twenty-five years.

In fact, of course, all of our experiences, if we are helped to reflect upon them, become an integral part of our learning. The long years of depression and anxiety were to give me an insight into the world of the trapped and desperate, which I could never have obtained from books.

One of the tragic things about mental illness is the shame people feel at being depressed or anxious or psychotic. Looking back, I can hardly believe the shame I felt and the certainty that revealing my illness would lead to my dismissal. As things turned out, I had no need to reveal it at work because fate intervened to change my life yet again.

24

RETURN TO CHILE:
1992

I n February of 1992 I went to Birmingham to be interviewed for the
BBC's *Woman's Hour*. Afterwards, I was approached by a producer
who asked me if I was interested in taking part in a radio series
about revisiting past experience. It was as though a bell rang in my
head and I answered before I could think: 'It would have to be Chile.' As
I said it I knew that such a trip would be way beyond their budget: but
apparently it wasn't and the man said he'd be in touch. I don't remember
what I thought then, but later on I knew that I must accept, for such an
invitation might never come again and I would be crazy to refuse the
opportunity to confront my demons once and for all.

Looking back, this decision to revisit Chile clearly had a major impact
on me, augmenting the anxiety which was never far below the surface of
my mind. About a month later I went to Ireland to lecture in Galway. The
day before the lecture I visited the leadership team of the Columban
Fathers in Dublin to ask them what they thought about my proposed visit
to Chile and whether or not the BBC producer and I could stay in their
Santiago house when we went to Chile to make the programme. I think
that at some level I was hoping that they would say no so I could grace-
fully call the whole project off, but they were kindness itself and said that
we would be welcome to stay at the Santiago Centre House, the official
headquarters of the Columbans in Chile. I left there both pleased and
terrified; this visit to Chile was really going to happen and who knew
what might become of me.

It was on the train to Galway that I experienced my first (and, mercifully, my only) panic attack. I was sitting quietly in my seat, reflecting on
the events of the morning, when I began to feel desperately giddy once
again. My heart pounded and I wondered if I was about to have a stroke.
I had a powerful sense of impending catastrophe and was deeply afraid.
I'm not sure how long it lasted: I remember wanting a cup of coffee but
not daring to get up from my seat lest I fall to the ground. I felt a terrible
sense of loneliness too, because, although surrounded by people, I dared
not tell anyone how ill I felt. Eventually, we arrived in Galway and I
greeted my hosts as though nothing had happened. That night I gave a
public lecture and I can remember clutching the edge of the stage before
I ascended it, certain that I was going to fall over.

Clinical anxiety frequently accompanies depression and, in my experience, it is more difficult to deal with. Depression brings low mood, guilt,
low self-esteem and lack of energy, but anxiety makes one deeply afraid
of all manner of things and also of nothing in particular. I know now that
I was afraid of returning to Chile: I thought that I would once again be
taken by the Secret Police, tortured and possibly killed. Curiously
enough, I didn't know it then; I just knew that I felt dreadful from time
to time and my sleep was more disturbed than ever.

Around this time, I sought help from Mike Snelson, the psychiatrist
whom I had first met in 1984. After we had met a couple of times he
decided I should begin antidepressants and put me on a small dose of a
drug called clomipramine. Initially, as so often happens, I felt worse –
giddy and peculiar and confused – but I battled on, giving a fundraising
talk for the hospice on the Thursday, a lecture at St Anne's Hospice in
Manchester on the Friday, a Day of Recollection at a London seminary on
the Saturday and an interview for a TV programme on the Sunday! I'm
not sure exactly when I started to feel better: most antidepressants are
said to take six weeks to be fully effective, but I know that I started
sleeping better within a few days. The pills made my mouth dry and my
bowels constipated but that seemed a small price to pay for being able to
sleep.

For the previous ten years I had slept only four or five hours a night,
sometimes only two. Suddenly the nightmare was over. I no longer felt
anxious and I no longer had insomnia; it all seemed too good to be true.
After a week's holiday in France I carried on as before, working flat out at
the hospice when I was there and lecturing when I wasn't. In June I went
to Italy for two days with John Newbury from the BBC, a Methodist
minister who was at that time a member of the BBC's religious broad-

casting team and the person designated to accompany me to Chile and tape record my reactions for radio.

The purpose of our journey was to meet with Father Bill Halliden, the Columban Superior in Chile at the time of my arrest. John taped an interview as Bill and I reminisced about the day of my arrest and I remember feeling desperate at the memories and wanting to hide under a duvet with my latest teddy bear. I survived, of course, and we returned to the UK and I took the sleeper back to Plymouth in order to work (and lecture!) the next day.

At the beginning of July I took two weeks' study leave (I was allowed three each year) to attend a course on spiritual direction in North Wales. I knew that this was not strictly medical education but reckoned that, as spiritual care was an integral part of my work with the dying, it was a legitimate use of my time. I enjoyed the course enormously, but three days before the end I received a telephone call from the hospice chairman requesting my presence at a meeting on the Sunday that I returned home. He refused to discuss the reason for the meeting and my anxiety levels rose. Eventually, I said to him, 'I need to know if the sword of Damocles is hanging over my head.' My memory is that he said cheerfully, 'Maybe it is and maybe it isn't.'

On the Sunday afternoon, therefore, after the six-hour drive from North Wales, I presented myself before the chairman and another member of the hospice Council and was informed that the Council had decided that the post of Medical Director should be full time, that is, five and a half days a week rather than the four days that I had negotiated after the Council decision in 1984. At first I thought this was another attempt to clip my lecturing wings, but it was made clear to me that my contract was being terminated and that they proposed to advertise for a new Medical Director.

So that was that: I'd always been afraid that I'd be sacked and now it had happened. At first I was deeply angry, but more than anything I was frightened. In three months I would be jobless, and what would I do, what would happen to my home when I could no longer pay my mortgage?

With hindsight, I do not blame the hospice for dismissing me because I see now that, although I never took time off that was not legitimate, I took it in such a sporadic fashion that it was disruptive to the smooth running of the hospice. I know too that my lack of interest in management issues was unhelpful because senior members of staff inevitably have management demands made upon them and I mostly turned my back on these. My sadness and anger at the time stemmed from the fact that I was given no warning that the Council were unhappy with my performance, but perhaps I was more difficult to talk to than I realised and they did what they thought was best for the hospice.

As it happened, what was best for the hospice turned out to be best for me too, because my colleagues in the hospital created a job for me and I was appointed to bring the skills of palliative care into the hospital setting, a role in which I was enormously happy for the next three years, after which I was allowed to concentrate fully on providing for the emotional needs of the hospital's cancer patients and their families. More of this later.

In the second week of November 1992, I returned to Chile after a gap of seven years, ostensibly to make a radio programme for the BBC, but mainly to confront my demons: the memories of torture and imprisonment and the terror which had accompanied it. I took three weeks' annual leave and spent the first week with friends in Florida, after which I was joined by John Newbury and we flew to Miami and thence to Santiago. At an intellectual level I knew that Chile was once more a democracy and that there could be no threat to my life, but at a gut level I was deeply afraid. I thought that there must be members of the security forces or the government who resented my endless human rights testimony and would leap upon me in some dark alley. The reality of my visit was very different.

On arrival at Santiago's Pudahuel airport I passed through immigration without any comment being made and was suddenly enveloped in a wonderful group hug of friends old and new. The leader of the welcome party was New Zealander Father John Griffin, the then superior of the Columbans in Chile. With him was my friend Jane Kenrick of the Sisters of Mercy, now working with AIDS sufferers in Valparaiso, and a number of other religious, men and women. John and I were carried off to the Centre House and made more welcome than I would have believed possible.

Within minutes we were shown the scars on the house resulting from my arrest. First was the bullet hole in the dining-room wall and a memorial photograph of Enriquetta, the Columbans' maid, who had been shot. The most dramatic for me, however, were the bullet holes in the fridge, which was still functioning seventeen years on. The bullets had entered the fridge door and ricocheted inside it, tearing larger holes in its interior. I knew then how lucky Bill Halliden and I had been because we had been hiding under the kitchen table only a few feet from that same fridge.

During the next few weeks John and I sought to retrace the steps of my Chilean adventure. My first stop was in the Calle Bilbao 285, but my house had gone, demolished and replaced with a petrol station. It was a curious feeling to look where my home had been: my life with Consuelo and the chows. Jane Kenrick came up from Valparaiso and with another Columban friend, Father Alo Connaughton, we visited the Villa Grimaldi, the torture centre, and Tres Alamos, the massive detention camp where I had spent nearly eight weeks. The Grimaldi was empty, locked and barred, but painted on its walls were amazingly beautiful and forthright words and images naming and commemorating those who had suffered and died within. At a lunch party with around fifteen of my former prison companions I heard that there were two proposals for the Grimaldi: one that it should become a park of peace and the other that it should be sold for housing. Incensed, I wrote a letter to the President, requesting that it should stay as a place where people could remember their dead. I received no answer but the park was made and I revisited it on a subsequent trip nine years later.

Two of the most heart-warming reunions were with the Jesuit priests Fernando Salas and Patricio Cariola, who had asked me to treat Gutierrez. The last time I had seen them had been in the military court where they had both been in leg irons. They were both well and engaged in their separate ministries, grateful no doubt, as I was, to be alive.

After meeting with the women with whom I'd been in prison I met again with Gladys Dias, the reporter and MIR activist who had been so badly treated by the DINA. She came to the Centre House and inter-viewed me for a magazine for which she was now working.

After we had fulfilled our obligations in Santiago, John and Jane Kenrick and I took a little holiday in Chile's beautiful south. We travelled overnight in a wonderful old train, sleeping in polished mahogany bunks with velvet curtains. After a lovely dinner and a good night's rest we alighted in Talca, one of Chile's southern cities. There I met with Bishop Jorge Hourton who had been the head of the Catholic Church's Vicaria (Diocese) of Solidarity, formed the day after the DINA closed the famous Comite de la Paz, the Committee for Peace, which had banded together medics, lawyers and others in the early post-coup days to help those people in trouble with the DINA. Bishop Hourton had published a message of farewell to me after my deportation, a brave act in those days of repression and persecution.

After Talca, we travelled south again to see the lake country and I bought some local wool which I later knitted up into a sweater. I have a wonderful photo of John and Jane and the owner of our hotel busy winding the wool into balls. We had a riotous evening as the woman told us all of her adventures during the coup. After a couple of nights in the south we returned to Santiago and, after many warm farewells, John and I flew back to Miami. I then returned to my friends in Fort Myers Beach, while John took his precious collection of tapes back to London.

After another week I returned to the UK and my work at the hospice. I have few memories of the weeks leading to Christmas and my last days at the hospice. My 1993 diary tells me that I had a farewell party with the nurses and doctors on 3 February; I know that I had flatly refused to accept the charade of a final meeting with the Council and I chose my own farewell present – a designer teddy bear whom I named Jeremiah.

Two weeks later I launched the new department of palliative care at Plymouth's Derriford Hospital with a lunchtime lecture at the Medical Centre on 'Emotional Distress in the Terminally Ill'. As one door closes, another opens and, for me, this was the beginning of an exciting new decade.

25

CARING FOR THE DYING
IN THE HOSPITAL:
1993

After a tedious period of searching for an office in Plymouth's
Derriford 800-bed general hospital, I was offered a room on the
haematology ward by Dr Archie Prentice, the senior haematologist. I was allowed part-time secretarial support and persuaded
Barbara Tappy, one of my two secretaries at St Luke's to make the half
hour journey across the city three or four times a week to help me
organise a palliative care service in the hospital. I was given a completely
free hand: no one else in the hospital claimed any expertise in palliative
care so no one told me what to do or snapped at my heels in any way.

After the intense atmosphere at the hospice I rejoiced in the freedom
of hospital life. My first task was to decide what, as a single-handed
doctor, I could offer to this enormous community of doctors, nurses and
patients. In the beginning, I thought it would be advice, support and
education for the doctors, especially the juniors, and made sure that each
ward had my office phone number. The referrals were initially slow in
coming but once the word got around that I was available, I had a steady
flow of requests to see terminally-ill men and women, mainly on the
surgical wards.

It took me a while to realise that what I *thought* I had to offer was not
really what was wanted. I had imagined that the junior doctors would be
anxious to learn from me how to talk with the dying and how to ease

their pain and other symptoms. I couldn't, however, have been more mistaken. It was the nurses who called me because they knew that their patients deserved better care than they were receiving but they didn't know how to implement it. Although I assessed each patient carefully and recommended any changes in medication that seemed appropriate, the most important part of my work turned out to be talking and listening to people.

Before I go any further I should make it clear that the patients I saw were not 'mine' to do as I wished with: they 'belonged' to the consultant under whose care they had been admitted, so that I could suggest a particular course of action but not implement it. This was not necessarily a problem, for I was familiar with the British system and, provided I was polite and diplomatic, few feathers were ruffled. I took great pains to record my findings, thoughts and advice in the patients' notes but, looking back, I know I should have written to each consultant after I had seen their patient. If I had done that, the profile of my work would have been raised throughout the hospital and I would probably have got on better with the consultants, both in general and in particular. Unfortunately, I didn't see it that way at the time. Instead of power dressing like my colleagues and lunching with them in the doctors' dining room, I did my own thing sartorially and ate lunch quietly in my office. Politics has never really been my thing!

I did, however, manage to do some very good work with individual patients. On receiving a referral, I would go to the ward and speak to the nurse in charge, who would then refer me to the nurse who was responsible for the individual's care. It was usually this nurse who had instigated the referral and she would tell me that Mr or Mrs X was suffering from terminal cancer and seemed distressed or confused. When I asked the crucial question, 'How much does she know about what's happening?', the nurse would look blank and say to me and any listening colleague: 'Well, I *think* she knows, but she doesn't talk about it. What do *you* think?' I would then ask about the patient's family and usually found that they had been seen by the doctor and 'knew the score'.

After this initial conversation with the nurses I would go off to the office with a cup of tea and the patient's notes to acquaint myself fully with his or her situation. This frequently took an hour or more as I waded through thick folders, reading the endless copies of consultants' letters and struggling to understand the house doctor's hand script. Key to this exercise was a meticulous examination of all X-ray reports, scans, blood tests, operation notes and histology findings. I had to know, before I saw the patient, what sort of cancer he or she had, how it had been treated, what stage it was at and whether there was any further treatment possible. Only then was I ready to see him or her.

Ideally, I should have taken the junior doctor with me, but I soon learned that they were (genuinely) too busy to spend as much time as it took me to medically assess and psychologically 'counsel' a patient. I found, too, that junior doctors, like their seniors, were more interested in cure than in care and they did not attach the importance to palliative care that I and other hospice professionals did. This was not, of course, true for all the junior doctors: some of them cared deeply about their dying patients but they too were burdened by pressure of work and the lack of life experience that is inevitable in youth.

I saw the patients, therefore, on my own and always in privacy, refusing point blank to discuss death and dying with other patients listening in behind the curtain. Over the weeks and months I learned on the job and honed my people skills with each encounter. First, of course, I would introduce myself as having been asked by their consultant to talk to them and then I would ask if they would mind telling me the story of their illness. Mostly, patients were only too happy to tell the tale of how they had been well and then, either suddenly or gradually, became ill. Each story was unique but almost all contained the same elements of worry, disbelief, fear, anger and sadness. There was worry when serious illness was suspected, disbelief and then fear as the diagnosis was confirmed, anger when people were treated shabbily and sadness when their condition did not improve. I heard stories of good GPs and bad, of kind consultants and arrogant ones, of hopes raised and hopes dashed, but most of all I heard tales of obfuscation, of the prevalent culture of the conspiracy of silence. This was 1993: twelve years after my induction into working with cancer patients, and speaking the truth was still a problem. True, doctors were no longer lying but they were still steering clear of their painful obligation to 'break the bad news' to those who were going to die.

There is something enormously powerful in listening to a fellow human being's story of suffering, whether it be in the hospital or in the psychotherapy consulting room. The problem in the hospital, of course, is lack of time: everyone is *so* busy that they are mostly unable to give people the time they need. At that particular time, however, I was my own boss and could allocate my resources where I felt they were most needed. During the forty-odd minutes it took a patient to tell me his story I was able to give him my full attention so that he felt, perhaps for the first time

in his illness, truly 'heard'. I was able, in this way, to establish a relationship of trust, so that when the moment came to ascertain what he knew
about his illness and its prognosis, I was able to speak the truth in a
manner that he could accept. For many patients, my visit provided confirmation of what they knew in their hearts: few men can lose weight and
strength, see their family in tears and their doctors embarrassed without
realising that things are not going well. Once they know the truth,
however, most individuals find that they have inner resources that they
would never have believed possible: I cannot recall a single man or
woman who lost his or her dignity in this situation.

The listener, of course, must be comfortable with the person's tears and
be able to preserve a loving silence as the patient wrestles with his
emotions. Occasionally, patients had no understanding of the seriousness
of their condition and were devastated at the news that their illness was
terminal. I found these situations personally very costly because there
might be repercussions from the patient's family or the consultant. In
fact, however, I have no memory of regretting telling the truth because it
is the greatest gesture of respect that we can pay someone we are caring
for. This does *not* mean, of course, that doctors have the right or
obligation to force the truth on those patients who do not wish to be told.
When a patient said that he or she did not understand what was
happening, I always asked, 'Would you like me to explain things to you?'
Most said 'yes' – but a few people looked this way and that without
replying, so I would then retreat, with the suggestion, 'Would you rather
take things one day at a time?' This gave them unspoken permission to
put off facing the future until they felt ready.

During these three years I developed considerable skill in one-to-one
encounters with patients but I had yet to learn how to relate to their
families with equal sensitivity. I had, of course, spent many hours talking
to families at the hospice but they, by and large, had accepted that their
loved ones were going to die. Mostly they were impressed by the care
given at the hospice and deeply grateful for what we were all doing. In the
hospital, however, relatives of the dying often felt very differently. Only
recently aware themselves of the terminal nature of their loved one's
illness, they were often determined to 'protect' him or her by withholding
the cruel truth. 'We mustn't destroy her hope,' was the cry, 'she'll give up
if you tell her she's going to die.' This is the conspiracy of silence at its
most primitive: the desire to protect a loved one from pain. There is also,
I suspect, a shadow side to this desire and that is to protect oneself from
the pain of talking about death with those one loves. When my father was

dying it never occurred to me to tell him the truth. Would he have wanted to know? I've no idea, but perhaps if I *had* told him we might have had the most important conversation of our relationship. Who knows?

Some years later I did a nine-month introductory course in family therapy and it was only then that I came to understand and be fascinated by what is known as *systems theory*. A *system* is a grouping, for example the solar system or the eco-system, of objects or people in relationship with each other. A family constitutes a system, as does a team of colleagues at work. When an outside event impacts upon one member of the system, that person or object impacts upon the other members, who in turn act upon each other. A classic example of a family system under-going change is when a daughter reaches puberty. A previously peaceful and ordered household is thrown into flux: daughter rebels, father is angry, mother upset, younger children distressed, and so on. Each person in the family is affected by the change and each in turn acts upon the others. Puberty is bad enough but at least most parents anticipate it. Cancer or motor neurone disease, however, is *not* what we expect and when a family member is hit by illness there are major repercussions. This is particularly the case when the sick person is a parent of school-age children: suddenly the principal carer or perhaps the major breadwinner is ill. The well partner is frightened and often angry, sleep is disturbed, income is threatened, people are irritable, and so on. Each family there-fore has its individual drama along with its own habits, myths and beliefs: it is no wonder that the families of the terminally ill need a sensitive approach!

The very first thing they taught us on the family therapy course was how to draw and think about a family tree. After that I constructed one with each new patient and thereby learned not only who was around in their life but also who had died, gone to Australia, and so on. The key information to be gleaned from a sick person's family tree is who is there to support them and who depends upon them. The mother of small children is clearly vulnerable when hit by a serious illness, the single mother even more so.

Once I had gathered this information from a patient I was much better equipped to meet his or her family and understand who was who and what their feelings were about their relative's illness.

I make no apology if this chapter reads somewhat like a palliative care textbook: illness and death are universal phenomena and the more we understand about why patients, families and carers behave the way they do, the better we will be able to cope ourselves and help those whom we love.

Towards the end of 1993, my first year at Derriford, I was asked to vacate my room on the haematology ward and was given instead an office in the oncology department at Freedom Fields Hospital, some twenty minutes' drive from Derriford. The hospital there was to be demolished but oncology could not be moved for a further three or four years as the new department had not yet been constructed.

The business manager of the oncology unit at that time was David Bullivent, a man with enthusiasm and energy to improve and expand our service. He mentioned to me one day that he would like to develop a cancer support centre for the department because he had been impressed by these services in other units. He explained that a support centre was a place where patients could meet with staff and volunteers to talk about their fears and worries about having cancer. As he spoke I saw that such a centre could bring to the hospital the warmth and hospitality which we had generated at the hospice. Without further thought I said to him: pay me for three more sessions (half days) a week and I'll set it up for you. And so it was that the first seed of The Mustard Tree was sown, a venture which was to grow and flower beyond my wildest dreams.

26

───∽◦◡◦∽───

THE MUSTARD TREE:
1993

The Mustard Tree, like the hospice, had humble beginnings. David Bullivent authorised the refurbishment of the sitting room of ward 18, the vacated ward in which I had my office, and a group of us brainstormed as to how to staff it. Eventually we decided that the centre should be open all day, five days a week and should be staffed at any given time by two people – a member of the clinical staff (a nurse or radiographer) and a volunteer. The idea for the name was mine and came from the gospel parable of the mustard seed, 'the smallest seed of all', which grew into a tree and 'sheltered all the birds of the air'.

As I check my Bible for the accuracy of my quotation I am struck by the realisation that this is one of the images Jesus used to explain the Kingdom of heaven to his disciples.

> He put another parable before them: 'The Kingdom of heaven is like a mustard seed which a man took and sowed in his field. It is the smallest of all the seeds, but when it has grown it is the biggest shrub of all and becomes a tree so that the birds of the air come and shelter in its branches.' (Matthew 13:31–32)

When I was at Ampleforth having my Scripture lessons I anguished endlessly about what this phrase, 'the Kingdom of heaven', really meant. Like so many of the images in the Bible, you cannot say 'it is this' or 'it is that', but it occurs to me now that the Kingdom must be quite simply where

God is manifest as love and justice. I think now of the ancient Latin hymn, '*Ubi Caritas at amor Deus ibi est*', which translates as 'Where charity and love are dwelling, God is dwelling there'. I know that love was present like the wheat among the tares at the hospice and our vision of The Mustard Tree was that it too would be a place of unconditional acceptance, loving hospitality and patient empathic listening.

The other parable of the Kingdom that sheds light on the purpose of The Mustard Tree is that of the yeast: 'He told them another parable, "The kingdom of heaven is like the yeast a woman took and mixed in with three measures of flour till it was leavened all through"' (Matthew 13:33).

Looking back over the years, I believe that the impact of both the hospice and The Mustard Tree is not confined to those who visit it as patients. We are modelling a way of caring, a way of being with sick people, which hopefully, little by little, influences the way patients are treated throughout the hospital and the community.

In the early days, as one might expect, we had few takers and eventually most of the professionals involved in being physically present wearied of their inactivity and disappeared back to their various jobs. The one person who stayed, however, and who shared our vision was a woman called Sue Smith, and she gradually took on the role of centre manager.

I had known Sue ten years before when she was a bright and efficient senior radiographer working on the radiotherapy treatment machines. In the 1980s, she had been forced into early retirement by ill health. In 1993, Sue and I met again and, when I found that she was unemployed, I persuaded her to help us as a volunteer.

When it became obvious that she was needed full time, and was well enough to return to work, Sue did a management course and told us that if she was to stay we would need to pay her. Determined that the project should not go under, David managed to find the money to pay her and Sue became the manager of The Mustard Tree, a post which she holds to this day, twelve years later. That this was an inspirational appointment will become evident as my story develops.

It wasn't until I began deliberately to recall events of the period that I realised that ward 18 had become a veritable crucible of invention and new life that was to change the face of cancer care in our region and beyond. Around July of 1994, the department appointed two senior nurses to act as clinical nurse specialists (CNS). This was a development in nursing pioneered in the USA in which experienced practitioners were appointed to act as a resource, a role model, leaders and educators to the other nurses in their field. This vision has been an enormously successful one and now exists not only in oncology but in other specialties as well.

The two nurses appointed were Sian Dennison, a ward sister from the Royal Marsden cancer hospital in London, and Tony Shute who had worked in the Plymouth oncology unit for many years. Sian and Tony were the first clinicians to join me on ward 18 and they shared a small office round the corner from my own where they kept their own counsel and planned for the future. This was the first time I had encountered such independent nurses and my nose twitched with curiosity as to what they were up to.

Not long after Tony and Sian's arrival we were joined by Elaine Price, a former school teacher who had trained as a counsellor and was employed to provide a service to the oncology patients. There is no doubt that I got off on the wrong foot with Elaine, excitedly telling her what I thought she should do rather than enquiring what her plans were. After that first meeting, she too kept her own counsel and I fretted that I was not privy to her ideas.

Most of the time, however, I was far too busy lecturing to worry about what my colleagues were doing. Looking back over my engagement diaries for 1994 and the years that followed, I see that I was lecturing several times a week both in Plymouth and around the country. In between these engagements I began to train as a counsellor, persuading the course trainers that I was so experienced in listening that I should be allowed to join the second year. At the end of the year, I received my diploma in 'person-centred' counselling and felt that at least I had the most basic qualification in psychological care.

I see now that I was gradually changing the focus of my clinical work from the care of the terminally ill to those patients who had only recently begun their 'cancer journey'. This happened because I was no longer located within the larger hospital and my referrals for palliative care diminished. The Mustard Tree, however, was an ongoing source of patients worried about their illness and its treatment and I warmed to the task of trying to meet their psychological needs. Little by little, ward 18 became a centre of psycho-social care and I found that I had embarked upon a new career.

Towards the end of 1995 the opportunity presented itself for me to train as a psychotherapist and I entered upon a two-year course of training in cognitive analytic therapy (CAT). This involved weekly visits to Bristol, and, ever enthusiastic, I persuaded three friends to join me on the course. We travelled together each week, to meet with our tutor, a Buddhist scholar and psychotherapist called James Low, who was part of the psychotherapy department at Guy's Hospital in London. James was a superb teacher and seemed to enjoy his time with the Plymouth group as he supervised our casework. Once a month we had a training day when the various supervision groups came together for lectures and seminars. Most of the other trainees were experienced mental-health workers, psychiatrists or psychologists. Somehow, however, we held our own and all four of us passed the exams at the end of the two years.

By 1996, The Mustard Tree was flourishing and Sue had persuaded Macmillan Cancer Relief to fund a new state-of-the-art support centre to be built at Derriford attached to the new oncology department. By this time The Mustard Tree was able to offer a number of complementary therapies in addition to its basic work of listening and information-giving.

Early that year a friend and colleague of mine, Dr Jenny Lovett, was appointed as hospital consultant in palliative care, along with two specialist nurses and a secretary. These posts were also funded by Macmillan who had pledged their support for the first five years on the condition that the hospital took over the funding of the project when that time had elapsed. Initially, I had thought to apply for the medical post but I was persuaded by David Bullivent that I would find it too confining so I set my sights on becoming a psycho-oncologist with a qualification in CAT.

I should explain that a psycho-oncologist is a professional specialising in the psychological care of cancer patients and there were no members of the species south of Bristol. All the psycho-oncologists I knew were clinical psychologists or psychiatrists but as the specialty was in its infancy there were no qualifying exams which I was obliged to take before I could call myself one.

As 1996 ran its course the date approached when we should move the oncology department lock stock and barrel to Derriford. To help our fledgling department of psycho-social care prepare for life at the new hospital, David Bullivent brought in Jude Squires, a management consultant, to work with us in the hope that our various conflicts might be ironed out before the move. The worst of these conflicts was between Elaine and myself for, despite our common expertise and aspirations, we were quite unable to work together. The group met about six or eight times during the six months prior to the move but nothing really shifted and Elaine and I maintained a cordial dislike of each other until she left some years later. A colleague who knew us all told me that she had come to the conclusion that we each gave so much during our work with the patients that we had nothing left to be nice to each other. It's worth mentioning that ours was not the only conflict in the department as two if not three of the consultants had a hearty dislike for one another.

On 14 February 1997, the entire oncology department – doctors, nurses, radiographers, physicists, secretaries and ourselves – moved to a brand new department at Derriford, the largest hospital in the South West. I was given an office alongside the consultants and Sue had hers in the new Macmillan Cancer Support Centre, known by all of us as The Mustard Tree. The new building was beautiful beyond our wildest dreams. It was large, light and airy, with skylights and French windows opening onto a terrace. There were rooms for everything: a kitchen, two counselling rooms, two therapy rooms and a large 'activities' room for craft work, meetings, classes and the like. The main room was like a hotel foyer, with three groupings of sofas, chairs and coffee tables so that several different groups of patients and volunteers could talk together out of earshot of each other.

In such a beautiful setting, the work of The Mustard Tree flourished and, by the time I retired in 2002, there were around five hundred patients attending the centre each month. The complementary therapies have remained popular and soon included massage, reflexology, spiritual healing and meditation. The other aspect of the work that increased was the provision of patient information about the various cancers. We were able to provide an array of booklets, and in recent years Macmillan has funded the post of information officer, which is shared between two professionals, a radiographer and a nurse.

As the volume of work increased, Sue took on more staff: another Sue to staff the desk at the entrance and deal with the statistics, and Pat Stapleton, a delightful widow from Northern Ireland who trained as a massage therapist and reflexologist. Pat is now one of the key clinicians in the centre, listening for hours to the distressed and providing a link between The Mustard Tree and the wards.

A psychologist colleague, Tony Carr, who ran the university course in clinical psychology, once said to me, 'Design your service to be needs driven', by which he meant, find out what the patients' needs are *before* you create your service lest you waste precious resources on what isn't needed. I took this message on board and tried always to discern what was needed and respond to it.

Tony and I and hospice social worker Carolyn Brodribb worked for several years on a research project trying to meet the needs of the bereaved relatives of those oncology patients who had died. The initial idea was mine but as usual I wearied of the administration required and drifted away, leaving Carolyn and Tony to finish the project. Although the research findings were not earth shattering, the project developed into a free-standing service for those bereaved people requiring specialist counselling. The Plymouth Bereavement Service still flourishes, despite withdrawal of part of its NHS funding. Tony and Carolyn have trained generations of bereavement counsellors and supervised their work until Tony's untimely death from motor neurone disease in 2005.

Meanwhile, I was a free agent in The Mustard Tree and, to maintain my links with the oncologists, I offered to work one morning a week in the outpatient clinic which specialised in the treatment of women with breast cancer. I came to enjoy this work enormously and I learned first hand how difficult it was to be patient and empathic with only a few minutes to allocate to each patient. As time passed, I became more and more aware of the disruption the illness caused to the lives of the younger women with children of school age and I considered how we could respond better to their needs. The project which followed was for me the most exciting and rewarding of anything I had so far undertaken and it was to flourish for the next ten years.

27

❧───❧

FIGHTING SPIRIT:
1996

'Fighting Spirit' was the name I gave to a group programme for young women with breast cancer. It arose out of the desire of a small group of younger patients to meet others of the same age also wrestling with the disease. Of that first group, one was a 29-year-old single mother with a two-year-old daughter; another was in her thirties, happily married and the mother of two small boys. The rest of the group were also young mothers and were mostly under forty.

I modelled the group on the work of Fawzy and Fawzy, a Los Angeles psychiatrist and his wife Nancy. They worked in the John Wayne Cancer Center and ran groups for both breast cancer and melanoma patients. The Fawzy model was a psycho-educational one: a programme structured to provide both education and emotional support for the patients. The group was 'closed', in that once formed no further members were admitted, and small, that is, no more than eight women, so that the women could form a close-knit unit and, hopefully, come to trust each other. The group was also 'time limited' – it was limited to eight weekly two-hour sessions, although the group members were encouraged to keep in contact and support each other once the group proper had ended. During the course of ten years, Kathy Smeardon, my co-facilitator, and I ran over twenty groups and worked with around a hundred and twenty women.

The first group began at Freedom Fields and was held in a small private house, an annexe to the oncology department. After we'd got to know each other, I asked the women to hold a brainstorming session in order to come up with a list of subjects they wished to be informed about. In addition to wanting further information about breast cancer and its treatment, they wanted to know more about diet, exercise, the impact of their illness on their children and, lastly, how to make a will.

From the very beginning, these young women tore at my heartstrings. They were so brave and so determined to survive, not for their own sakes but for that of their children. They were so open, too, about their difficulties, and ready from the outset to be friends with and look after each other.

Young breast cancer patients are very suitable for groups of this nature for several reasons, the first being that, provided the cancer has not spread beyond the axillary (armpit) lymph glands, they all have a chance of survival. The treatment, too, is relatively uniform, consisting in most instances of surgery, chemotherapy, radiation therapy and hormone treatment. To put it crudely, these women are subjected to a greater or lesser degree of mutilation of their breasts, six months of drug treatment, which makes them vomit and (possibly) lose their hair, five-times-a-week hospital-based radiotherapy treatment for six weeks and, finally, hormones designed to bring their reproductive lives to an end for five years, if not for ever. It is no wonder, then, that these women have so much in common or that they need help. We calculated that most women completed treatment in about twelve months, if you take into account the time elapsing between one or more episodes of surgery, six months of chemotherapy and six weeks of radiotherapy. It was in some ways a year of their young lives lost and Fighting Spirit was designed to mitigate that loss and help the women cope with their situation.

All the groups except the first were held in the activities room of The Mustard Tree. Sometimes we sat in a circle in comfy chairs but if I arrived before Kathy, I invited the women to sit around a large oval table, which to me felt like a farmhouse kitchen scenario. It was useful, too, when I wanted to draw diagrams to explain things and especially at break time when we shared coffee and cake.

From the beginning, the groups were informal in that we called each other by our first names and Kathy and I were at pains to wear our authority lightly. We tried to make the experience as unstressful as possible and introduced ourselves as women like them, with strengths and weaknesses of our own. On the first day, we asked the individual women to introduce themselves, to tell us about their families and then, when they felt comfortable, to tell the story of how they discovered they had cancer.

This last exercise was the most taxing and some women broke down and wept as they spoke of their fear and the psychological pain involved in facing a mortal illness. When a woman cried another member of the group would leave her seat to comfort her; as each realised how much they had in common with the others, the bonding was palpable. After everyone had told their story, we took a comfort break and replenished the teas and coffees. At the first session, I would provide a feast of whatever food I had in my office – biscuits, fruit cake, chocolate – and ask if someone else would provide the refreshments the following week. This simple role-modelling of hospitality set the tone for sharing and each week a different woman brought cake or fruit or whatever she felt suitable.

After the break, during which the women chatted among themselves and Kathy and I exchanged views on the group process, we met together again and brainstormed what people wanted to know. In the first group I had brought in a number of 'experts' to teach on the various topics but that proved too difficult logistically, so I taught the women myself and gave them various handouts to take home. My co-facilitator Kathy is a nurse teacher and I realised that we were running the groups in much the same way as we had run our seminars for nurses on the care of the dying. The principle of the educational element was to empower the women by helping them understand their illness and its treatment. Many of the women were professionals: school teachers, nurses, radiographers (as well as those who were full-time mothers), and they were extremely interested in the information we gave them.

After the sessions on cancer and its treatment I gave them the basic information on nutrition supplied by the hospital dietician. There are many different 'cancer diets' put forward by various 'holistic' therapists but we stuck to the evidence-based more orthodox teaching. Once we had covered the most pressing items on the agenda, we encouraged the women to talk about their relationships with family members and with their doctors, both GPs and consultant surgeons and oncologists. As a psychotherapist in training I was fascinated to hear the different ways that the patients and their partners coped with the trials of illness. Quite a number of the husbands clearly found talking about their wife's illness with her extremely difficult and, although they were helpful in practical issues, they were bad at providing the emotional support the women needed. Some men, of course, took the challenges of the illness in their stride and were able to provide all the support needed.

Another interesting issue was how the women's mothers reacted to their daughter's illness. Some were wonderful – comforting, reassuring and providing practical help – but others found the possibility that their daughter would pre-decease them desperately threatening and demanded more support than they gave.

The women's accounts of how their children coped with their illnesses were often extremely moving. I remember the 29-year-old's toddler asking whether mummy's 'booby' would grow back. Occasionally we would have a woman in the group who'd developed breast cancer while feeding her baby and realised how difficult it was for both mother and child when she couldn't cuddle him or her because of recent surgery or radiotherapy. We came to understand, too, the enormous difficulties experienced by the single mothers with cancer if they had no relatives nearby. One woman related how, the day after her chemotherapy, feeling like death, she took to her bed, only to be asked by her seven-year-old son, 'Mummy, why are you so lazy?'

Although the subject matter of our conversations was deadly serious, the manner of it was often lighthearted. The women rejoiced in black humour as a coping strategy and often told jokes against themselves. The indignity of wearing a prosthesis was a frequent source of humour, especially when we organised a swimming session in the hospital therapy pool. One young woman was a photographer and decided to produce a book about the impact of breast cancer on women like herself.

The reader may question why we chose to work with the younger age group when all ages of women suffer from the disease. We were well aware of the difficulties of older patients but felt that the need of younger women to be with sister rather than mother figures had to be honoured. It was, of course, a question of resources: we simply did not have the time and money to offer the group experience to all the patients. We found, too, that women in their sixties had less interest in joining the programme.

Another category of patients that challenged us was that of the women whose disease had spread beyond the limits of their lymph nodes. Statistically speaking, these women were incurable and therefore in a very different category from the patients we chose to work with. We did, in fact, run two groups for the women with metastatic disease, and they worked reasonably well, but there is no doubt that the groups were 'heavier' and more difficult to run as a time-limited programme. One of the breast cancer charities runs a telephone support group for women with metastatic disease and I can see that this might work well. If I were to run such a group again I would make it both 'open' and continuous as the patients' need for support would increase as the disease progressed, in contrast to the potentially curable women whose need for support usually ended soon after their treatment was completed.

When the group ended we suggested that the members exchange phone numbers and keep in touch if they felt like it. Although some chose to put the group experience behind them, many women stayed in touch and had regular meetings to socialise and support each other. It was particularly moving when one member of a group developed recurrent disease because each woman knew that, there but for the grace of God, went she. As time passed, some women died and, in many cases, their fellow group members attended the funeral – an act of enormous solidarity and courage.

Over the ten years during which I ran the groups, I came to know some of the women really well. It was particularly hard, therefore, when they developed recurrent disease and eventually died. Sometimes they came to me with the news and sometimes I had to tell them that the X-ray or scan which we had so hoped would be clear was in fact indicative of disease which had spread. There was one young social worker, Annie, mother of two small boys, who seemed to be doing so well until she developed a swollen gland in her neck. The gland was hard to the touch, which meant it was likely to be malignant, but we still hoped against hope that her disease could be contained. On the Friday afternoon a week or so after a series of scans, she asked me if there was any news. I knew that I should not meddle and should wait for her to be told the results in clinic, as was the custom but it seemed so cruel to make her live with the uncertainty over the weekend. I phoned the bone scan and the ultrasound departments genuinely expecting that the news would be good, only to find that she had widely disseminated disease in all her bones and also in her lungs and liver.

The hard part was that she looked so well and her only symptom was a dry cough. It was *so* cruel: she was young and bright and full of life and loved her work and her family, and it was my job to shatter her hopes and rain down grief and despair on those she loved. It's no wonder that doctors used to lie to their patients about their prognosis. I spent the next two to three hours helping her assimilate the harsh truths of what was happening to her. When she had composed herself, she phoned her sister and then asked her husband to come to the hospital bringing the boys with him.

I sat with those boys in The Mustard Tree while she talked to her husband on his own, and then she told the boys that she was ill again. Eventually, the family left and I sorted out my papers and went home.

Another young woman, 'Barbara', who lives on in my heart, came from the depths of Cornwall and was referred to me for counselling because she had become depressed. One evening as we finished our session I worried that she might take her own life and, rather than send her to the psychiatric unit, I persuaded the sister on the oncology ward to give her a bed for a couple of nights. At first all seemed well but then at ten o'clock that evening I was phoned by the night nurse with the news that my patient was about to discharge herself and drive home to Cornwall.

It was a foul night and I considered my options as I drove to the hospital. If Barbara chose to discharge herself I could not stop her unless I got her 'sectioned', that is, held against her will because she was a danger to herself or others. I decided that the risk was insufficient and I must try persuasion. Eventually, after sitting on her bed for half an hour, I left Gus, my teddy bear, as a sort of hostage and promised that he would look after her until the morning. As soon as I had handed Gus over, Barbara disappeared under the bedclothes with him and, after a while, I decided it was safe to go home.

When I visited the ward the following day she and Gus were still hidden under the blankets but they soon emerged to greet me, slightly dishevelled but none the worse for their night together. I decided that Gus had better stay with Barbara until she felt better, so the two of them went off to Cornwall to look after each other. A week or so later, Gus arrived back in a brown paper parcel, muttering grumpily about the inadequacies of Royal Mail.

Even as I write this story I realise that I need to say a few words about bear therapy in general and Gus in particular. I was a child of the Second World War and although my mother gave me a doll and made various soft toy animals for me, I never had a bear. True, my elder sister's boyfriend Peter gave me a large plush bear from Paris but he was very hard and not really very huggable. I never owned a bear until my early fifties when I bought myself a small yellow one at Heathrow Airport on my way to Rome. Although I had an intuition then that this bear had magical qualities, it wasn't until I did my back in that I realised how great its powers were.

I was still at the hospice, still stressed and plagued with pain in my back, when one particular morning a kindly nurse offered me a massage. I lay on the couch as she applied the oils, relaxing as well as feeling rather guilty that I wasn't actually working. After ten minutes or so my masseuse decided she would try her hand at psychotherapy and started to ply me with questions about my private life. Irritated to be thus interrogated, I said firmly, 'Thank you, Jenny, I think I'd better get back to work,' and made to sit up. Halfway from the horizontal to the vertical position, however, I was seized with the worst pain I'd ever experienced (Chile included) as my back muscles went into violent spasm. I cried out in pain, Jenny panicked and ran for help and I lay on the couch in humiliated agony. After a cooling-off period of an hour or so I was still unable to move, so my colleague Mary called an ambulance and I was carried off to hospital on a stretcher while the patients watched in amazement.

Although I tried to be brave and dignified, I was very frightened, sure that my spine was collapsing and that I was riddled with bone cancer. As I was carried out to the ambulance I asked my secretary to go to my house and bring me a nightgown, a book and my bear. Imagine, therefore, my distress a couple of hours later when Christine arrived with the *wrong* bear: one with no magical powers at all! Too embarrassed to send her back to my house, I thanked her and lay miserably awaiting the worst. At nine o'clock that night, however, help arrived in the shape of my good friend Carolyn, the hospice social worker. With tears in my eyes, I said pitifully, 'Carolyn, I need my bear.' Carolyn, bless her, understood and, after I had explained to her just which bear it was, went off with my house keys to fetch it.

For the next two weeks I clutched that bear as if my life depended on it. If it fell off the bed I courted the ire of the nurses by ringing the bell for them to pick it up. Later, when I was on the mend I risked life and limb by hanging over the side of the bed to rescue it. From that time on, I knew that I needed a bear to protect me.

The bear was, of course, what the child psychotherapists call a 'transitional object', something which links the child with its 'secure base', its home and carers. Just as the child endows its piece of blanket with magical powers of protection, so I had endowed my bear with similar properties. From that time onwards, I never went anywhere without a bear. The original one was replaced by Abraham, who some time in the late 1990s was replaced by Gus.

After a while I started taking Gus to work with me and when someone in the Fighting Spirit group was upset the bear would be passed to her for comfort. When patients were in grave distress I sometimes gave them a bear of their own to keep and explained that it would only protect them if they gave it the power. During my years at the hospital, Gus went to work with me every day and I took him onto the wards when I went to see patients. I'm sure the male consultants thought I was deranged but they were too polite to say so. Now that I am retired and have two real live teddy bear-like dogs, Gus too has retired but he still comes with me when I go away for the night. When not actively on duty, he lives on my bed or the sofa, ready to spring into action if needed.

My final bear tale takes me back to the year 2000 when I found myself invited among the great and the good to take lunch at the Mansion House as a guest at the Lord Mayor of London's millennium luncheon. As it happened, I arrived back from lecturing in Australia on the day of the lunch, so I went straight to the Mansion House, as high as a kite on sleep deprivation and jet lag. As I left my coat and luggage at the cloakroom I decided to check in the bears (Abraham and Humphrey), but the young woman in charge dissuaded me and I took them with me.

It was a very grand do and I recognised various politicians of note. Eventually there was a sort of traffic jam on the stairs leading to the dining hall and I found myself wedged in a sea of pin-striped suits. Keen to be sociable, I enquired of the man next to me, 'Have you brought your bear?', at which he spluttered nervously, 'No, was I supposed to?'

My next encounter was with a tall man carrying a bright green card, so I asked him what it was for. He grinned and said, 'I'm a member of the band!' It was only when I arrived home in Devon that I discovered that I too had a green card and that it was a personal invitation to meet the Queen! What Her Majesty would have made of Abraham and Humphrey we will never know. The tall man, I found out, was the Deputy Commissioner of Police. As I said, it was a very grand do!

28

∽⌇⌇∽

JEREMIAH'S JOURNEY: 1995

As I explained earlier, when I left the hospice my friends asked me what I would like as a leaving present and I chose a teddy bear: not just any teddy bear, you understand, but a handmade, mohair *designer* bear who cost around seventy-five pounds. He was a rather short-sighted individual so I bought him a pair of gold-rimmed spectacles and named him Jeremiah after the Old Testament prophet. Some weeks later, while on a shopping spree in nearby Totnes, I revisited the bear shop and bought Jeremiah a wife, whom I named Rebecca; later still I acquired two children, Sam and Sophie, so that Jeremiah and Rebecca's union might be fruitful.

One Saturday morning when I was due to help my friend Kathy teach a group of nurses about grief in children, I felt inspired to write a story and in the space of a couple of hours I put together 'Jeremiah's Story': the tale of a bear named Jeremiah Frisby, his wife Rebecca and three children, Sam, Sophie and baby Chloe (whose arrival I have omitted to mention). The story began, as all good stories do, with 'Once upon a time'. 'Once upon a time there were two bears, a very short-sighted gentleman bear called Jeremiah and a lady bear called Rebecca. Now Jeremiah was a very clever bear who spent long hours each day studying, while Rebecca was just the opposite. She was a friendly, light-hearted little bear who loved life and people and all sorts of fun . . .'

The story goes on to tell how one night when Sam was about eight,

Sophie, four, and Chloe, eighteen months, the two Frisbys were sitting talking to their good friend Finbar, who, like Jeremiah, was a don at Balliol College, Oxford. As they were talking, Rebecca suddenly cried out, 'Oh, my head! My head,' and then fell to the floor in a dead faint. Finbar sent for an ambulance and Jeremiah called in their cleaning lady, Mrs Racketts, the raccoon, to sit with the children while he and Finbar went with Rebecca to the hospital.

Alas, for the purposes of my story, Rebecca dies of a brain haemorrhage and Jeremiah becomes so depressed that he can barely look after the children. Meanwhile, the children manifest their grief in their own ways, Sam by playing truant from school and Sophie by clinging to poor Mrs Racketts, who took over the children's care. At last, Finbar insists they see his friend Rufus, the grief therapist and, little by little, the family are helped to come to terms with their loss.

'Some months after Rufus's first visit, on a hot August afternoon, Finbar arrived bearing three large packages. The children clamoured round him and, like a magician, he produced his gifts. For Sam, there was a marmalade kitten, for Sophie, a fluffy white rabbit, and for Chloe, a golden teddybear. Jeremiah spoke: "Do you know, Finbar," he said, "I do believe we're going to be all right."'

The story was a great success and our teaching session buzzed with speculation about the effects of the loss of a mother upon a young family. From that day on the Frisbys took on a life of their own and Jeremiah, Rebecca, Finbar and the children were called upon for all teaching on child bereavement. It was obvious, therefore, that when a group of us decided to institute a programme to help grieving children it should be called 'Jeremiah's Journey'. I should explain here that we were not the first to start such a venture, nor were we the first to adopt a bear as our hero. Julie Stokes, a bright young clinical psychologist with hair like a Botticelli angel, started 'Winston's Wish' at the Royal Gloucester Hospital after winning a Winston Churchill Scholarship to study child bereavement in the United States. Julie did her psychology training in Plymouth and spent several months on a placement at St Luke's, so we take great pride in her achievement and are quite ready to admit that she was our inspiration.

Julie's programme, which has been very successful, involved a weekend programme for the children and a parallel one for the grown-ups. The aim was to allow the children to meet with others who had also lost someone close and encourage them to think and talk about their loss. Their bear, Winston, was a mythical creature who understood the pain of grieving children, and each child was given a Winston bear to take home.

Jeremiah's Journey was born of identical aims: to reduce bereaved children's sense of isolation by introducing them to other grieving children, and to help them to think and talk about their loss. The spur to this endeavour was my encounter with young mothers dying from breast cancer or other tumours and the realisation that there was no provision of emotional support for the children they left behind. Initially I sought the help of a senior child psychologist but he was extremely busy and soon to leave Plymouth. Realising that if we wanted a service for these children we must provide it ourselves, I gathered together a group of like-minded professionals and discussed what we should do.

The people involved in setting up the service were Jacqui Stedmon-Taylor, a senior child psychologist, Di Maynard, a social worker in the paediatric unit, Ann Tucker, a nurse therapist working with children, and Helen Taylor, a primary-school teacher who had been widowed a couple of years before. We had no money at all but were each prepared to give our time gratis because we were convinced of the importance of the project. Realising that we did not have the resources to run a weekend programme like Winston's Wish, we chose an after-school group model in which the children attended weekly for six weeks, with their parents, for an hour and a quarter. Although the time we chose was quite brief, it was long enough for the children after a day at school and also long enough for us by the time we had prepared for the group, run it, debriefed and cleared up afterwards.

Right from the beginning the project worked well. Jacqui, Ann, Di and Helen worked with the children, along with David Lobb, my neighbour, and later John Wright, a social worker, while I worked with the parent groups, encouraging them to share their experiences with each other and talk about not only their personal grief but the difficulties they were experiencing with their children. The children's groups were play-orientated with an almost equal ratio of adults to children so that each child could be helped with their task at the same time. The high point of the group programme was the making of memory boxes – initially shoe boxes, but later, purchased hat boxes, which the children covered with glue and glitter, paper and feathers to their own design. The idea behind this was to encourage each child to remember and talk about the person they had lost.

The ages of the children varied from teenage to five years old and they were divided into two or three groups, depending upon their age. The teenage groups are always a challenge and are facilitated by an experienced member of the team. The first few groups were run in the annexe to the radiotherapy department at Freedom Fields hospital but after February 1997, when we moved to Derriford, we were able to use the facilities of The Mustard Tree, which were larger and more pleasant to work in.

After the move to Derriford the number of children referred to the programme increased and we decided it was time to employ someone to co-ordinate the project. Our first co-ordinator was Emma Snelling, an assistant psychologist gaining practical experience between her first psychology degree and her three-year training in clinical psychology. Emma, and the young psychologists who succeeded her, were a tremendous find, being young, enthusiastic, extremely intelligent and (amazingly) cheap.

Emma threw herself heart and soul into the work, combining assessment visits to referred families, data-base creation and fundraising without difficulty. We housed her and her computer in a claustrophobic, windowless room opposite the therapy rooms in The Mustard Tree so she had an instant hospital base and family with it. Although the hospital have never had any money to give us they have provided heat, light, telephone and IT back-up, without which we would have been hard put to survive. The first three years of the post were funded by a charitable trust and we have continued a somewhat hand-to-mouth existence with a succession of grants since then.

Emma brought into our lives the IT expertise of her partner John and the firm for which he worked, Bluestone. Before long we were a real organisation with our own headed writing paper, complete with Jeremiah Bear logo, information leaflets and collection boxes. Bluestone take care of our printing needs to this day and make the charity look very grown up, especially now we have our own website.

In addition to the groups, we have always run a number of social occasions for the children's benefit. A couple of weeks after the end of a group the team takes the children to Woodlands, our local adventure park, for a fun day: as Jacqui says, it's giving the children the message that it's OK to have fun, even when someone has died. Then there is the Christmas party attended by around a hundred children, most of the team, all the parents and of course Father Christmas, a magician or a puppet show and Jeremiah Bear himself. In recent years the outings have increased, including a picnic in the woods with release of helium balloons to which farewell messages are attached, and a special outing for the teenagers.

Emma stayed with us for two years before returning to the university to complete her clinical psychology training. She was followed by Vanessa and then by Lisa, also assistant psychologists, both of whom expanded and enriched the service. In particular they were full of energy and ideas for fundraising, arranging an annual Jeremiah's Journey auction and ball, a fun run and stalls at all local charity events.

Sometime during Vanessa's or Lisa's tenure we appointed an office manager in the form of Debs, who had lost her brother and cared passionately about what we were doing. Debs made the ultimate fundraising sacrifice by having her beautiful dark hair publicly shorn. Alas she was too shy to allow national exposure or we would surely have made a fortune. Lisa made her mark by organising the first Jeremiah's Journey charity shop, which has been a huge success bringing in around a thousand pounds a month.

Last in this line of co-ordinators is Joanne, the youngest of the group. In her early twenties, Joanne has an amazing gift with the children, and a boundless supply of patience and good will towards the slightly weary core team – still Jacqui, Di, Anne, Helen and myself. A great addition to our group of founders and trustees has been Pat Stapleton, who is assistant manager at The Mustard Tree. Twice widowed herself, she has enormous understanding of the difficulties of the children and their grieving parents.

My work is always with an adult group and we allocate the parents to one of the two groups at a planning meeting. We try always to group together those with similar experience: sometimes we have four parents who have lost a child, sometimes women who have lost their husbands to a violent death, whether accident, suicide or murder. These groups are often a very powerful experience, not only for the participants but for the facilitators as well. The first meeting in particular has to be very carefully handled because I try to get the individuals to speak a little about their loss. Although this is very painful for all it is an enormously powerful bonding experience for the participants as they realise that they are not alone in their grief.

Loss of a child is probably the hardest bereavement for a parent to cope with. We see losses from leukaemia and other childhood cancers, traumatic deaths and even suicide. Over the years we have worked with the parents of four child suicides, mostly hangings in the home by boys of eleven or twelve. In such situations it is almost impossible to know if the death was accidental or deliberate and the parents are torn apart in their grief and bewilderment.

The sceptical may wonder what good we can do with such deeply traumatised people in so short a time. True, wounds such as these take years to heal and are never forgotten, but the very fact of meeting another with similar pain is somehow helpful. We provide, too, a safe space for the bereaved to express their grief and, so often, their rage, at what has happened to them. The experts tell us that there is no way we can short-circuit grief: it is like a long dark tunnel which has to be navigated before respite is achieved. My job as a therapist is to work alongside such people, sharing their pain if I can. It is always a temptation to try to blot out grief with alcohol or drugs but such relief is only temporary and often bought at a terrible cost. I have watched in desperation for three years as a young mother of five has drowned her sorrows for her dead husband in alcohol, achieved no attenuation of her grief and done irrevocable damage to her children in the process. Many professionals have been involved in her care, but we are all powerless unless she stops drinking.

The other benefit to members of the adult groups is the opportunity to share their experiences of their children's response to grief. Until recent years it was commonly thought that children do not grieve as much as adults, and that they are 'resilient', 'getting over' their grief quickly. We know now that this is quite untrue: children do grieve as deeply as adults, but they manifest their sorrow in different ways. Many older children 'act out', that is, behave badly in response to their grief. They are rude to their parents, destructive in the home and cause trouble at school. They fight, play truant and neglect their school work, especially boys when they leave the relatively nurturing environment of primary school for the much larger secondary school where the other children and teachers may know nothing of their loss. Many bereaved children are bullied at school simply because they are different from the others. Celebrations of Mother's or Father's Day become a nightmare because they have to declare their loss.

Since Jeremiah's Journey started around ten years ago, we have offered a number of seminars for school teachers to prepare them to understand and help their grieving pupils. These teaching sessions have been well received, though it is always difficult for the schools to carve out time in a busy curriculum. Schools sometimes ask our help when a schoolchild dies, especially if it is a sudden death, perhaps a canoeing accident or other sports tragedy.

It is curious to reflect that in this age of advances in the treatment of physical disease there is still virtually no NHS provision for adults and children suffering traumatic loss. A couple of years ago Plymouth Health

Authority withdrew funding from the Plymouth Bereavement Service, which had been running successfully for over ten years. Jeremiah's Journey receives no state funding: we are entirely dependent upon charitable grants and local fundraising. We have recently decided to employ a part-time fundraiser to help Joanne, especially with the complicated grant applications.

At the end of each group we hold a simple ceremony of remembrance. We begin with my recounting the tale of how Jeremiah is sent by his children in search of Rebecca's spirit. Jeremiah goes first to Nepal to meet with the abbot of the Monastery of the Great Spirit who tells him he will find Rebecca's spirit in the Land where the Rainbow Ends. Jeremiah then embarks upon his Great Journey, travelling by hot-air balloon across the world until he finds a rainbow over the Great Australian Sandy Desert. Terrified, he parachutes from the balloon and lands in a thornbush in the desert. Here he is rescued by a little Aboriginal boy who takes him to the leader of their tribe, a wise old woman called Nancy. Jeremiah, still unnerved by his jump, pours his heart out to Nancy who listens carefully to him, then laughs a great belly laugh which reduces Jeremiah to tears. 'You silly old bear,' she exclaims, 'you won't find Rebecca's spirit at the ends of the earth because she is right there with you, wherever you go.' Jeremiah looks at the sun through his tears and there is the end of the rainbow right where he is. Jeremiah returns home and tells the children that Rebecca will never leave them because she lives for ever in their hearts.

After the story the groups convene for the last time and each person, old and young, is given a silver star on which they can write a message to the person who has died. The stars are then hung one at a time on a golden tree and each child is given a floating candle to take home. Lastly, each child receives a gift, a small teddy bear and a handmade velvet 'coping' bag containing symbolic coping tools: a piece of rose quartz to keep in their pocket and hold when they are sad, a notebook and a pencil, a worry doll and a dream-catcher to filter out the scary dreams. Then, after much hugging, the families leave and we, the team, heave a sigh of relief: another group programme has been completed. Two weeks later the families re-group for a fun day at Woodlands, our local adventure park.

A month or so later, the families are invited back to tell us how they feel about the group. We ask them, individually, what worked for them and what they would have us do differently. We have thus, over the years, fine-tuned the programme in response to the participants' feedback.

Unlike Fighting Spirit, which ended when I left Derriford, Jeremiah's Journey will surely continue because it gathers to itself an increasing number of healthcare and teaching volunteers who are determined that the grieving children of our city will be supported.

29

LEARNING TO BE A PSYCHOTHERAPIST: 1998

n January 1998, when I was sixty-one years old and four years from retirement, I embarked upon the second part of my psychotherapy training, a two-year course in cognitive analytic psychotherapy with a qualifying exam and a ten-thousand-word dissertation at the end. This would, if I were successful, secure me membership of the United Kingdom Chartered Psychotherapists (UKCP), the exclusive body which certifies bona fide therapists.

The first two years of my CAT training had been both exciting and fun as David, Viv, Carolyn and I made our weekly journeys to Bristol. The advanced course, as it was called, was a very different affair: it was much more demanding and required not only that I travel to London once a week for two years but that I arrange to have my own psychotherapy during the duration of the course. Carolyn and Viv had decided not to do the advanced course and though David also enrolled, he chose to travel up to London on the early train while I, unwilling to rise so early, travelled up the night before. Each Wednesday evening, therefore, I caught the six o'clock train from Plymouth to Paddington, arriving in London around ten. Once at Paddington I had to cross London to get to Guy's Hospital, near London Bridge, and collect the key to the nurses' home where I had arranged to stay. The nurses' home was incredibly bleak but the beds were clean and they provided tea-making facilities, so

I could not complain. Mostly, I saw not a soul as the nurses had long since gone and the rooms were used for the occasional overnight stay by a patient's relative or a passing foreign doctor. Most important, they charged only twenty pounds a night, so I felt I could justify my dinner on the train and a taxi across London when I arrived.

The following morning I was up at seven and hurrying to London Bridge station and the train to Tulse Hill where I had a fifteen-minute walk to the house of my CAT therapist, a delightful woman called Analee Curran. After my hour of therapy I walked back to the station and took the train to London Bridge where I bought a cappuccino and a raisin pastry, then made my way back to Guy's for two hours of group supervision.

Our supervisor was Claire Tanner, a shrewd and highly intelligent American woman from Colorado who had come to CAT via psychiatric social work. She worked part time in the eating disorders unit at the Bethlem and Maudsley psychiatric hospital, and spent the rest of her week supervising therapists or seeing private clients. I liked Claire enormously and was soon providing her with an Americano coffee and a cinnamon bun to sustain her during supervision. There were four of us in the group and we took it in turns to present our clients to Claire and the rest of the group. It was a very useful process, though I have to admit that I could only remember my own clients and got a bit lost with those of the other trainees.

We finished with Claire at 1.00 p.m. and were off again, rushing down Tooley Street to the Psychosynthesis Centre where the rest of our course began at 1.30. There were around eighteen of us – psychologists, an occupational therapist, doctors, nurses, and others without a healthcare background. I am not greatly at ease in large groups and made few friends other than Claire during the two years of the course. Most of the socialising went on during the supper break when the group went together to the pub. Exhausted by the lectures and naturally shy, I spent the hour's break wandering round an open-air market and having a solitary meal in an Italian restaurant. At 7.30 our eleven-hour day was over and I fled for the underground, desperate not to miss the last train to Plymouth. The journey home had little to recommend it as the train was always packed and I was hard put to find a seat, let alone revise the day's notes. I arrived home after midnight hoping against hope that my car would not have been stolen or vandalised in the station car park.

Any reading or other course work had to be done at the weekends as the rest of the week I was occupied with my hospital work. Little by little, however, I absorbed a proportion of what they tried to teach me and, when the time came to sit the exams, I passed. I did my dissertation on staff relationships and conflict in the development of our psycho-social oncology service and, to my amazement, got a credit. The whole enterprise was a mammoth effort and at the end of the course in December 1999 I vowed never to go to London again!

The following year I was invited to give a series of lectures in Japan on the psychological and spiritual care of cancer patients and persuaded my hosts that, as I had no husband or wife, they should pay for my niece Lucy to accompany me. To my delight, they agreed and on 15 July we flew from Heathrow to Osaka and then took the bus to Kyoto. That first night in Japan was amazing as our visit coincided with an eclipse of the moon and the streets were full of young people in traditional dress clattering over the cobbled streets in their wooden shoes.

My first lecture was in Osaka, the second in Nagoya and the third in Tokyo. How much the audience understood I shall never know but they had a translation of my teaching material, so at least they could read it later. Our hosts looked after us well and struggled manfully on Lucy's behalf to find her vegetarian food. Lucy ventured out shopping on her own and, to my delight, bought me a baby's kimono and pantaloons for Gus who was looking distinctly conspicuous in his American Osh Kosh jeans.

After a week in Japan we flew to Shanghai, a very expensive add-on to the trip as there seemed to be no cheap flights between Japan and China. As we drove from the airport I was amazed at the skyscrapers, buildings unlike any I had seen before. After two days at Shanghai's famous Peace Hotel we flew to Wuhan to begin our five-day cruise down the mighty Yangtze Kiang River. This was truly the experience of a lifetime as we passed through the famous Three Gorges and visited the construction site of the dam which was to change the Yangtze and those who lived along its banks for ever. It was this trip through the heart of China which gave me a sense of the immensity of its population, for we passed city after city whose populations, I was told, were in the region of five million. We made frequent stops and our tour guides took us to displays of theatre, silk factories and, of course, all manner of temples. My souvenirs, a terracotta mother and child, a jade horse and an original painting of the three gorges, are daily reminders of an amazing journey.

I have been so lucky over the years because my gift for teaching has taken me round the world more than once. One of the most heart-warming trips was to lecture in Concepcion in the south of Chile, where I was welcomed for my professional expertise rather than my renown as a prisoner of conscience. I have also revisited Australia a number of times to lecture to various healthcare or pastoral audiences and have had great fun during halfway journey breaks in Bangkok, Bali and Singapore. One of my favourite places, apart from South East Asia, is Capetown, where a lecture trip led to my meeting Stephanie Kilroe, a vivacious mother of three who was for many years the chief executive of Life Line, an outreach project providing counselling and support for women in the townships. Steph is now one of my dearest friends and I have stayed with her many times.

In 2001 David Lobb and I embarked upon what turned out to be one of the most ambitious and taxing ventures of my career: we organised a CAT psychotherapy course in Plymouth. This was a 'practitioner course', a two-year training to equip participants to practise CAT within their core profession. In the early days, David and I worked well together. We planned the curriculum between us, according to guidelines laid down by the CAT training board, and I persuaded Claire Tanner to come to Plymouth once a month to conduct a training day. David had worked hard to qualify as a supervisor and he was joined by Liz Fawkes, a delightful red-headed CAT therapist who travelled each week from Dorset to supervise the trainees in their case work.

My task was to run weekly seminars to supplement the monthly training days and I embarked upon them with my usual confidence, anticipating that I would be the success that I normally was in the rest of my teaching endeavours. My confidence, alas, was misplaced, and after two or three sessions I realised that some of the trainees were dissatisfied with my contributions. Looking back I can see that there were a number of contributory factors. The first was that David, Liz, Claire and I had been so busy getting the course organised that we had not spent time planning either the content or the format of the seminars. Left to my own devices, I embarked upon teaching in a didactic rather than an interactive style which is more appropriate for adult learners. After a few weeks we changed the format by selecting an academic paper to be read by all prior to the seminar so that we could discuss it as a group. I didn't particularly enjoy these sessions: I was tense and anxious and felt that the trainees were only moderately interested in the material which often felt dry and uninspiring. As time went by, however, I relaxed and became much more at home with some of the seminar group members, especially with the trainees who were new to psychological therapy. Among these there was

Rachel, a teacher and mediator from Swaziland; Barbara, a practice nurse; Martin, a clergyman with a background in banking; and Justin, who worked in a centre for helping violent men.

After I retired in August 2002 I continued teaching, holding the seminars in my home. In this more relaxed atmosphere, with trainees with whom I did not feel threatened, the sessions became a delightful learning experience for all of us. There was also a group of psychologists from Cornwall whom I taught at home and with whom I felt more at ease than I had with their Plymouth counterparts.

With hindsight I see that my informal manner was not to everyone's taste, especially those whose training led them to expect a certain formality in professional endeavours. Little did they know that we had no secretarial backup and I spent hours on the phone with all manner of departments negotiating times and rooms for teaching. All in all, it was a valuable experience, but one which I have no wish to repeat.

Despite our various difficulties, the course was a success and Devon and Cornwall are the richer by seventeen psychotherapy practitioners.

In January of 2002 Claire Tanner and I went together to Australia. My invitation was to lecture to hospital chaplains in Tasmania and I was once again able to persuade my hosts that I needed a travelling companion and that Claire would be a great addition to their conference. We made our first stop in Singapore, staying with my friend Rosalie Shaw, a palliative-care specialist who teaches all over South East Asia. Rosalie, who is Australian, started her career as a nurse and went on to study medicine, specialising in palliative care. She and I met at a conference in Singapore in 1982 and have been good friends ever since.

After a night with Rosalie, Claire and I flew on to Bali, my most favourite stop-off on the route to Australia. Ignoring the beach resorts, we went straight to the famous arts and crafts village of Ubud where we stayed at the Tjampuhan, an idyllic hotel which I knew from a previous visit. Ubud is a shopaholic's paradise and Claire and I spent a happy day browsing among the paintings, carvings and textiles for which Bali is famous. The Tjampuhan is set on a steep hillside with terraced gardens that are a blaze of colour with tropical flowers. Claire and I luxuriated in the pool and indulged ourselves with beauty treatments and massage.

After forty-eight hours in paradise we flew to Melbourne to visit my friend Rosemary: art critic, teacher, group facilitator and so much more. I first met Rosemary in my final year at boarding school where, as Sister Mary St Thomas, she taught me art and listened to my adolescent worries. Now, fifty years on, Rosemary is still a Sister of Mercy but lives alone and worked at the university. She is enthusiastic and knowledgeable about Aboriginal and contemporary religious art and has mounted a number of exhibitions in both Canberra and Melbourne. Rosemary is one of my most favourite people: warm and gracious, witty and wise, she is a powerful witness to the ability of religious women to flower and grow outside of a formal community. After three days with Rosemary and a brief meeting with other friends we flew to Launceston in Tasmania, where the pastoral care conference was due to open that night.

For four days I lectured on the psychological and spiritual care of the terminally ill, answered questions and made friends with the chaplains while Claire too lectured and socialised. On the last day we flew back to the mainland of Australia and on to Sydney where we spent one night with another school friend, Ann Long and her husband Geoff, and a mutual friend, Catherine Grey.

The Longs are both doctors, retired now but passionately involved in ecological issues. Their architect children have built them a marvellous house in the depths of the bush, about two hours south of Sydney, where they are in daily communication with kangaroos, wombats, kookaburras, lyre birds and all manner of other indigenous flora and fauna. Catherine lives and works in Sydney with her psychotherapist husband Brian.

By the following evening we were in Bangkok at the Marriott Riverside Hotel where Claire was reunited with her husband Arthur who had flown out to join us on the last stage of our holiday. Bangkok is on the Chao Phya River and I love staying in one of the many hotels built along its banks. Part of the joy of lecturing in Australia is dipping briefly into the exotic culture of South East Asia on the way home.

We returned to the shock of a bleak English winter, and the endless coughs, colds and flu which are endemic in our hospitals. Surveying the wall planner in my office I realised with a jolt that there were just six months before I retired and my thirty-nine years' service in the NHS would be over.

I had given little thought to retirement, living as I did in my extremely busy world of the here and now. The training in psychotherapy had been not only to equip me for my psychological care of cancer patients, but also to provide a professional interest and, hopefully, a small income when I had finished at the hospital. I suspect that, for some people, approaching retirement is a bit like dying: they face the inevitable and then carry on in denial as if nothing is going to change. Others, of course, can't wait and cross off the days of their calendar with glee while they dream of cruising the Mediterranean or visiting the Galapagos Islands!

My dream was very different: I would buy a golden red chow puppy and call him Anka, as a symbol that my travelling days were over and I would thenceforward be happily anchored in Plymouth where I would see my psychotherapy clients and write lots of books.

30

GAIN AND LOSS:
MAY–DECEMBER 2002

In May 2002 I spent a week in Canada, lecturing in Winnipeg on 'A Spirituality for the Long Haul' to a group of doctors, nurses and clergy. I had never realised before how flat the mid-west of Canada is, having previously visited only Montreal and Vancouver, and found the city without charm. To my amazement, however, I discovered they had their own ballet company, so I took myself off to see *Carmina Burana* on the first night. My various lectures went well and I returned home to an afternoon of lecturing at the hospice followed by a session with a psychotherapy client. The bonus of the trip was a two-day stopover in Montreal with my friends John and Clare Hallward, whom I normally see only during the summer in Maine. The Hallwards are among my dearest friends. We first met in Plymouth in the early 1980s when John sought me out after having read *Audacity to Believe*, the book about my Chilean adventures. The story he tells is that the Archbishop of Canterbury, Donald Coggan, was preaching in the cathedral in Montreal and mentioned my book in his sermon. The owner of the cathedral bookshop rushed out at the end of the service to find the few dust-covered copies of *Audacity to Believe* in his basement, one of which was bought by John.

Just a week after my return from Canada, 18 May was a red-letter day, marking as it did the beginning of my new life as utterly besotted dog owner. Anka, thus named because he was to anchor me to Plymouth, was just ten weeks old when Kathy drove me to Bugle in Cornwall to pick him up. All puppies, of course, are adorable, but Anka was something else. Chow puppies are a ball of red golden or black fluff with big paws, tiny ears and a face which looks like that of a teddy bear. How I could have imagined that I could combine work with motherhood is still a mystery to me. On the Monday morning I took him to my outpatient clinic, where he was made much of, and then to the hospice where I was lecturing in the afternoon. My students and the nurses were enchanted, but alas the management was not and I soon received a letter asking me not to bring him to the hospice again. Personally, I think that visits from a puppy would be just what the hospice doctor would prescribe for her patients, but alas there had been a previous visit from an unclean dog which had infected the hospice cat and cost the management the earth in vet's fees. I remembered Teddy the collie who had lived at the hospice and given endless pleasure to both patients and staff and thought how times had changed.

Life went on. Anka grew apace: by mid-June he was fourteen weeks old and almost too heavy to lift. When I was at work he spent time with my Canadian neighbour Dorothy in the flat above, where he would sit on the balcony and watch the world go by on Plymouth Hoe. The CAT course was in its second year and I continued to teach my four seminar groups. The rest of my time was spent as usual seeing patients in the breast cancer clinic, running my last Fighting Spirit group, and teaching here, there and everywhere. Suddenly, on 7 August it was my last day: my 39-year career in the NHS was over.

That evening, my friends in The Mustard Tree held a party for me and I duly presented myself, with Anka, now twenty-two weeks old and in part my gift from my friends, as the guest of honour. I am not a great party lover, but this was different. Strung high up in The Mustard Tree was a banner which read SHEILA CASSIDY: THIS IS YOUR LIFE, and sitting in a great circle were my niece, Lucy and a myriad of friends with whom I had worked over the past twenty years. There was John Brindle, my first boss in the oncology department and the man who had created a job for me in the hospital when I left the hospice. Then there were Lucy, Jenny and Caroline, the three Macmillan nurses with whom I had first worked at the hospice. From those far-off days also came Christine and Barbara, my two secretaries, who had supported me so loyally over the years. Knowing that I had neither husband nor lover, they quietly became my family, doing my washing when I was ill, driving me to the station when I was off lecturing, filling my fridge when I returned from a trip and covering for my absence when they thought I would get into trouble.

When I left the hospice, Barbara chose to come with me and drove that extra ten miles or so to Derriford each day without complaint. For the first year, we shared an office – the side ward on the haematology ward – and then, when I moved to the vacated ward at Freedom Fields, we each had our own space. Barbara is truly a woman without guile, loved by her family and all her workmates, and without her my ten hospital years would have been much the poorer. (I was able to take her, with Lucy, to Australia on one of my lecture trips, by exchanging a club-class ticket for two economy ones.) Along with Pat and Sue from The Mustard Tree was Carolyne Brodribb, a close friend since hospice days. Lastly, there were Lisa and Jacqui and other friends from Jeremiah's Journey. It was wonderful to see how many people had come to wish me well in retirement – I suddenly knew myself truly loved.

When the story of my life had been told and various gifts presented, Anka and I made our way home. Luckily, there was a parking space outside my flat, and, even more luckily, a young man with what I took to be naval bearing just happened to be walking down the street. Never a woman to miss the chance of assistance with carrying heavy things, I enlisted his help and gained an unexpected friend. John Garner was only thirty when we met, but as he is an old-fashioned sort of man, the age gap seems of no consequence. At the time we met, John lived just three doors down the street from me, in a wonderfully elegant first-floor apartment with two balconies overlooking the sea. His father Martin is a clergyman, a widower, whose wife died of breast cancer in 1998. John has an identical twin, James, another brother, Phillip, and a sister, Penelope, who lives in Tavistock, not far from Plymouth. I have gone into some detail about the Garners as John has become my closest friend over the past three years and also, at times, my lodger. Our casual friendship took on a new turn when I invited him to Christmas lunch after his car broke down en route to his father on Christmas Eve. By the time my family arrived for lunch, John was ensconced at my kitchen table cleaning the silver, an activity which immediately earned him the title of 'the butler'!

Within two days of my retirement, I flew to the USA for my annual holiday with John and Clare and whichever of their children were visiting. Anka went to spend the two weeks with Lucy and Harry, where he blotted his copybook daily by barking whenever he was shut outside in the garden and chasing Lucy's grey tabby cat who is not named Crazy Claws for nothing.

The moment I arrived home, I was off again to lecture, first to Derby, then Glasgow and finally Birmingham and Oxford. My whirlwind of activity came to a sudden halt – on 29 October, when I found out that I had breast cancer.

The diagnosis took me completely by surprise. I attended the hospital for my regular mammogram examination, expecting to rush off after it to give a seminar to a group of CAT trainees. So used was I to the procedure that I lay quite peacefully waiting for the doctor to come and tell me that all was well. I was quite stunned, therefore, when she came in and informed me that I had a malignant tumour in each breast. There followed a series of biopsies, during which I wept quietly because of the pain and, worse, the worry that Anka wouldn't understand if I died.

When it was all over, I went off to join the CAT group and the following day returned to see the surgeon for the results of my biopsies. Roger Watkins, one of the three breast surgeons, was kindness itself, but there was no way of softening the blow that I had a malignant tumour in each breast. By the time I saw Roger I knew that I wanted both breasts removed. Roger was shocked and said there was no need as the tumours were small: less than one centimetre in diameter. I was, however, adamant. I had been on hormone replacement therapy for fifteen years and I calculated that, if there were two tumours, there could be other cells waiting to turn malignant. Any recurrent disease following a lumpectomy (removal of the tumour only) is usually prevented by a six-week course of radiation therapy but I dreaded the possibility of even minimal reduction in my lung capacity as my asthma had diminished my exercise tolerance since I was a child. Roger agreed rather reluctantly to perform the operation and we set the date for two weeks hence, on 13 November.

I had always thought that if I ever became seriously ill I would keep the information to myself and pretend that nothing was amiss. To my great surprise, however, I found that my instinct was to be completely open with everyone – friends, family and colleagues alike. The hardest people to tell were my family because, of course, they were the most deeply affected, but telling friends and people at work proved to be a powerful coping strategy. Each person I told asked me what they could do, so I placed orders with everyone for flowers and chocolate so that my house was filled with beauty for the month following my operation. The two weeks until my surgery passed quickly as I had my usual teaching commitments – though how I concentrated on lecturing, I can't recall.

On Monday 11 November I was called to attend the hospital at 8.45 a.m. to be seen in the pre-admission clinic and got my first taste of what it was like to be a patient under the new bed-saving regime. The 'clinic' was an office where I was interviewed by a nurse who wrote down my medical details and then I was sent off to have various tests done. First, there were the blood tests in the blood-letting department, then the ECG in the cardiology department and lastly the chest X-ray. I caused a ruffle of radiographers' feathers by asking that a radiologist should check my films before I went on my way. I knew it could be done because I'd seen a radiologist I knew passing by but I wasn't to know that my films were mildly abnormal so they had to be compared with my previous films before an opinion could be given. The previous films, of course, were in the X-ray store which happened to be five miles away, so I had to wait a couple of hours before the radiologist rang me at home to tell me that I was not riddled with lung secondaries from my tumour.

Two days later, at 7.30 a.m., I presented myself for surgery, armed with Gus my bear and a large bag of knitting in case I had to wait. I was to be nursed in a side ward on one of the surgical wards, so, after such an early start, I was looking forward to lying on my bed snoozing or reading my book. I could not have been more deluded! The ward secretary said she was sorry but there was no bed for me, so would I please wait in the day room with the other new admissions. I was not amused and even less so when I found that all the women were accompanied by their husbands and there was an overpowering smell of cigarette smoke. I retreated hurriedly, unable to face polite conversation, and established myself in the corridor with my knitting where I could see what was going on in the ward. I should admit before I go any further that I probably brought this lack of welcome on myself because I had declined a bed on the breast cancer ward because I thought the beds were too close together. Little did I know that a few hours later I would be just *so* grateful for a bed on that same ward and that I wouldn't care at all about the closeness of the beds!

Three hours passed and it was still only 10.30 in the morning, and I was still knitting furiously. Then the ward sister approached me and said that she had secured a better place for us to wait. Still naively expecting to be put to bed by some friendly nurse, I followed the other women in pursuit of the sister as she led us through the hospital, clutching our overnight bags, teddies and other vital possessions. Eventually we arrived to find that we were now in the sitting room of the day-surgery unit where we were to wait until called for our operations. I returned to my knitting, longing for coffee and other creature comforts.

At around one o'clock I was asked to put on my hospital gown and dressing gown and a short while after that I was told that a nurse had come for me. Well, I thought, at least I can lie down on the trolley, but no such luck. The nurse apologised and said we were to walk to the operating theatre. Kind woman, she carried my overnight bag while I wrestled with Gus, a new bear who had been delivered to me an hour before and, of course, my knitting. Feeling distinctly sheepish in my dressing gown and slippers, I was grateful that we took the B route to the theatre, passing through diverse narrow corridors and a secret lift.

When I arrived in the theatre, however, I found that there was a reception committee of theatre nurses to greet me with hugs and a card: they were former students and Carolyn Brodribb's daughter-in-law Lisa who was a theatre sister. Suddenly it all seemed bearable and I chatted with the women until it was time to climb at long last onto a trolley. Then it was the needle in the vein, the counting to ten and I was away.

I was on the operating table around three hours and by the time I came round night had fallen. As my brain struggled to locate where I was, my hands went up to my hurting chest and found a layer of bandages and cotton wool. I knew then that it was true: I really did have cancer and they had cut off both my breasts. Gradually I became aware that there was someone with me and by a strange coincidence it was a woman I knew, Primi, a nurse who had worked at the hospice when I was medical director there. All I remember about that night is how safe I felt with Primi behind those curtains. Now that I really needed a bed I had one and, better still, I had a nurse I knew and trusted to care for me. With infinite gentleness, Primi washed me and then massaged my hands and my feet until I fell asleep once more.

In the morning, of course, she had vanished and when the curtains were drawn I found myself in a small ward with about fifteen other women. I realised then that I didn't need a single room and, indeed, I was better off with this strange sisterhood, all of the members of which were afflicted with the same condition as me. To my amusement, the woman in the bed opposite mine was one of my patients and she waved shyly at me. There was even a cordless phone especially for the patients, so whoever could walk would answer it and take it to the bed-bound. It was a good system. The nurses were kind and clearly knew what they were doing so I relaxed into being a patient as well as a doctor.

My friends came and went with flowers and bears and chocolate and I hung a wonderful yellow-orange cardboard sun sent by my friend Elizabeth in New Zealand. I was, I think, a good-enough patient except for the time a foreign doctor addressed me as Mrs Cassidy, to which I responded sharply 'DOCTOR Cassidy!' The man cringed and I felt a little guilty and said, 'Do call me Sheila: but I'm not a Mrs!' After three days they said I could go home, so I called my friend Jacqui and she, John her partner, Simone her daughter and I walked slowly to her car, laden with flowers, knitting, books, Gus the bear and all my other belongings. Jacqui stayed a while to make me tea but then she left and Anka and I were alone. I was glad to be home but it was quite scary to be so alone so soon after my operation. At about six, however, my friend Kathy the nurse teacher arrived and I felt safe and loved and cherished once more. Kathy stayed the night and the following day Pat, my sister-in-law, also a nurse, took over my care, so I was well looked after.

By the Sunday night, however, I began to feel feverish and unwell and the next week was one of the most unpleasant I have experienced. Pat took me to the hospital on the Monday morning but my surgeon was away and the doctor I saw said he could find nothing amiss. On Tuesday I felt worse but didn't like to complain too much, so on the Wednesday morning Pat left and I was once more alone. The moment the door closed behind her I burst into tears of self-pity and loneliness. Later on I pulled myself together and rang Carolyn to ask her if she would stay the night with me. She agreed readily, so I felt better at once and rang my GP's surgery to ask if the district nurse could visit.

She came at about three, cheerful and professional in her nurse's uniform and, after taking a brief look at me, snorted and said, 'You're toxic', meaning that I had an infection. Then followed long phone calls as she located the duty doctor, it being my GP's half-day off. The prescription arranged, she went off to collect it and returned triumphantly an hour later with the antibiotics. I swallowed the capsules eagerly and she went off, satisfied with a job well done. The next day, however, I felt much worse, sick, dizzy and extremely unwell. Thinking that the pills had not yet done their job I lay in despair on the sofa for the rest of the day. The next day was Friday and I still felt like death, so, unable to diagnose, let alone treat, myself I rang the surgery and asked my GP to visit. The receptionist was not best pleased but I stood my ground and an hour later I was telling my tale of woe to Dr Murray. Never have I been more impressed with or grateful for a doctor's ministrations, for he worked out that I was 'dying', not of an overwhelming infection as I had suspected but of the side-effects of the antibiotic!

Within twelve hours I was on the mend and although I had several more trips to the hospital for wound care, I never looked back. Ten days later, I forgot all about having breast cancer because Anka's half sister Mollie, a sturdy, short-legged, black chow bitch, came to stay.

Mollie was fourteen months old when she came for a two-week trial to see if she could settle in a new home. Her previous owner was a young widow who had four other dogs and was persuaded by the breeder to part with Mollie when I phoned to enquire if she had a black bitch. Mollie was, and is, a fabulously beautiful but extremely wild creature. She was distraught at being separated from her owner and paced my small terraced garden hour after hour looking for an escape route. After about three days she relaxed enough to lie down but it was about ten days before she would let me near her. She ate well, however, and got on well with Anka, so the breeder told me to persevere for the full two weeks and, suddenly, I had a new friend. Mollie is now my devoted companion, snoring under my high Victorian bed and warming my feet on the sofa when I take my afternoon nap. She remains, however, deeply suspicious of strangers and hates being touched by anyone she does not know. This latter trait makes our public walks quite complicated as she is extremely curious and likes to sniff people's legs which, if they are dog lovers, they take as an invitation to friendship, which, of course, it isn't.

Inside the house she is highly territorial and barks loudly at all strangers, especially tall men. Sometimes I wonder if she had a traumatic experience in childhood but I can only speculate as neither she nor her previous owner are telling! In the early weeks of our relationship Mollie did her best to get sent home, deliberately peeing on all the beds and both sofas. For a while I was desperate, for this was no territorial marking behaviour but a malicious emptying of a full bladder where she knew it would rile me most. Visitors were particularly at risk, so I never made up the spare bed until the last minute before bedtime. She was not, however, to be thwarted and the moment the duvet was in place would jump up on the bed and do her worst. I, however, was equally determined and bought pee-proof mattress covers for all beds and sofas, so at least she didn't wreck the mattresses and sofa cushions. After three months, she mercifully abandoned this form of protest and there have been no problems since.

31

◦◦◦ ◦◦◦

THE END OF AN ERA AND
A NEW BEGINNING:
2002

One of the things I used to notice about my retired colleagues was how well they looked and how relaxed and happy they seemed to be but it never occurred to me that I too could be well and happy and relaxed in my later years! At the time of writing this book I am sixty-eight years old, and I don't remember being so well or so happy for a very long time. It seems appropriate, therefore, to end this book by writing about the experience of being happy and peaceful in my heart.

Curiously enough, I don't miss my life at the hospital in any way. I greatly enjoyed the work I did but grew to hate the stress of rushing to be on time (not that I ever was!), making my way through the traffic and searching for somewhere to park. So, the first thing I enjoy about being retired is rising in a leisurely fashion and saying my prayers while I drink a cup of tea. Prayer for me continues to be important: a life-giving activity which, paradoxically, can be boring at the time. My discipline of prayer has changed over the years, according to my circumstances. For a brief period I prayed in the dark with a candle for an hour a day and wrote about it for a pious journal. But these days have long since gone and I now spend a very limited time in formal 'waste-of-time prayer'. Each morning I sit with my mug of tea and gaze out over the sea, opening myself to the Divine. Sometimes my mind is still, like a mountain tarn, at others it is invaded by thoughts of this and that. Sometimes a particular issue rises from the depths and I know what I should do about it; at other times nothing much happens. As Ann Lewin writes:

> Prayer is like watching for the
> Kingfisher. All you can do is
> Be where he is likely to appear, and
> Wait.
>
> From 'Disclosure' by Ann Lewin[1]

More often than not, Anka joins me on the sofa and demands that I scratch his back, so I have had to learn to pray while moving my fingers gently and rhythmically in his fur. I feel a bit like the Jesuit who asked the novice master if he might pray while smoking; I am simply responding to the instruction to pray at all times. When Anka and I sit on the sofa together, we face not the sea but the picture of my Dark Angel. This is an oil painting bought when the probation office down the road held a sale of work done by their clients. It would be more romantic if this was the work of a penitent old lag but in reality it was painted by the secretary. The picture shows the head of the angel, part of her wings and two hands raised – whether in dismay or benediction I am not sure. The face, wings and hands are dark against a glowing red-gold background and I have spent many hours wondering what sort of an angel she is. Angels, of course, are messengers and for a long time I thought she must be the bearer of bad news: of murdered girls, smashed motorcyclists and suicide bombers. More recently, however, I've decided she is a comforter so I send her each morning to look after the day's wounded.

For many years I had little use for petitionary prayer, convinced as I am that God has the whole world in his hands. Now that I am no longer actively involved in mending the broken and comforting the afflicted I feel the need to pray on behalf of the wounded presented to me each day on the various news bulletins.

Although my formal prayer ends when my tea is drunk, I am conscious of the Divine throughout the day, not continually of course but in sudden glimpses either in nature or in people encountered. Living, as I do, by the ocean I am ever conscious of God in the sea's changing moods. Each day I take my dogs down to the beach or, when the tide is high, we sit on rocks made smooth for sitting by Victorian Plymothians a hundred years ago. This is a particularly sheltered spot and I drink my coffee and bask in the sunshine, which in England is always received as gift, not right. My

Anglican priest friend Martin and I have christened this spot 'church' as I insist that I find God more truly present there than in my local parish services.

Perhaps this is the moment to come clean and admit that I have, for the moment (or perhaps for ever), given up going to church. There are many reasons which I could give but the most cogent one for me is the deep sense of God that I have in the world about me and a powerful conviction that Christianity is less about liturgy than love of neighbour.

One story is worth telling. Some years ago I went with a group of men and women on a sort of retreat-cum-holiday to Venice. I was the named retreat-giver and we were accompanied by a Catholic priest who was to say Mass. All was well until Father X (his name escapes me) made it clear to the Anglican members of the group that, though they were of course welcome to attend 'his' Mass, they could not expect to receive holy communion. I reasoned with him that this was a private liturgy and that, under such circumstances, surely there could be no objection to allowing these devout people to share the Eucharist. I told him that I had been at many private liturgies where the demands of charity overrode those of canon law. He was, however, adamant and I could only apologise to the group. Those affected by his implacable ruling were extremely upset and nothing I said was of any comfort to them. I tried to convince them that Christ was not bound by the limits of bread and wine and they had only to invite him into their hearts and he would be there. Alas, my theology did not convince them and I gave up trying. Each day at Mass I felt angry and deeply saddened for them and eventually decided to abstain from receiving the Eucharist myself in order to be in solidarity with them. I'm not sure that they even noticed but I felt that I was doing the right thing.

It may be that this experience was the beginning of my disillusionment with certain elements of Catholicism. Much later, my growing awareness of the abuse of children by both priests and nuns disturbed me at a very deep level. My anger and sadness was not so much with paedophile priests as with their superiors who covered up for them and the hierarchy in general who I felt should be more vocal in their penitence and their shame.

What angered me more than anything, however, was the abuse of children and pregnant girls by religious women. How, I reasoned, could these women who spent so much time on their knees be so cruel when they were working? One evening I saw a television programme about 'the Magdalens': the Irish girls who were sent by their families to 'The Good Sisters' to repent their illegitimate pregnancy and be cared for until they gave birth. This programme led me to buy the book *A Light at the Window:* the account of her time in a Magdalen home by midwife June Goulding. The account of the cruelty experienced by these unfortunate girls at the hands of the sisters made me sick with fury and shame. Of what worth was their daily Mass-going and other devotions if it did not shape them into loving, Christ-like carers?

These are difficult questions and I have put them to a couple of my priest friends. They too are deeply saddened that such cruelty could be spawned within the Church and they attribute it to the harsh religious formation of the young men and women who had entered the religious life with open, willing hearts. Hopefully modern understanding of psychology has put an end to such terrible corruption of young people. The paedophile issue, of course, is different and is likely to continue as long as there are men and women with a damaged sexuality.

None of the issues I've discussed are reason enough to give up going to Mass and I may well return to Catholic observance in the years to come. Meanwhile, however, I no longer believe it to be a 'mortal sin' to stay at home on Sundays and sixty-odd years of church-going seems enough.

The older I get, the more convinced I become that the essence of Jesus' teaching is about love of neighbour and not about sexual abstinence or religious observance. His message is summed up in these words from the Last Supper discourse:

> 'I give you a new commandment:
> love one another;
> just as I have loved you,
> you must also love one another.
> By this love you have for one another,
> everyone will know that you are my disciples.'
>
> (John 13:34–35)

The key question for all Christians, of course, is how do we live out that love for one another? My way has always been in caring for others in a professional but also a warm and loving manner. Now that I have retired from the hospital, I attempt to continue this 'ministry' as a psychotherapist. I see an average of two people each weekday in the comfort and privacy of my own home. Mostly, I see them not in my 'consulting room', which is rather dark, but in my living room where the sun streams in the French windows and the dogs lie peacefully at my feet. I have been practising as a therapist for eight or nine years now, if you count the four years of training, and the more I see people within this relationship the more spiritual an experience I find it. At an intellectual level, people and their relationships are infinitely fascinating, while at a human one it is a privilege to listen to people's stories and try to help them with their problems of depression, low self-esteem, loss or marital discord.

CAT – Cognitive Analytical Therapy – in which I am trained is a short-term, focused, highly collaborative psychotherapy which explores childhood experiences which have led to 'maladaptive' patterns of thinking and behaviour in adult life. The majority of my clients have suffered some kind of abuse in childhood, ranging from outright cruelty to psychological neglect. Sharing their story with a therapist and being respectfully listened to over a number of weeks can be a profoundly healing experience, though of course the more wounded people are, the more difficult it is to help them develop love and respect for themselves. As Philip Larkin says:

> They fuck you up, your mum and dad,
> They may not mean to but they do.
> They give you all the faults they had
> And add some extra, just for you.
>
> But they were fucked up in their turn
> By fools, in old style hats and coats,
> Who half the time were soppy-stern
> And half at one another's throats.
> From 'This Be The Verse' by Philip Larkin (1922–85)[2]

The psychotherapy brings me daily contact with all manner of people and, though tiring, feels a very good thing to be doing. It also provides me with a small income, which pays for my cappuccinos by the sea, the cleaning of my house and its windows, the milk and the dog food.

The source of my deepest happiness, however, is undoubtedly my dogs. Chows are highly independent, one-person dogs who are completely devoted to their owners. Austrian ethnologist Dr Konrad Lorenz believed that dogs are descended from two distant ancestors, the wolf and the jackal. He postulates that the jackals were tamed first and that when our forefathers began to settle in the arctic they encountered the arctic wolf and crossed their domestic dogs with it, producing an animal with close allegiance to its pack leader rather than the child-like dependence of the jackal dogs. Lorenz writes: 'The submissiveness of the childish jackal dog is matched in the lupus dog by a proud man to man loyalty which includes little submission and less obedience.' The other interesting fact is that, while jackals are carrion feeders, 'the wolf is almost purely a beast of prey and is dependent upon the support of his fellows in the killing of the large animals which are his sole means of sustenance in the cold season'. This latter observation confirms my experience with Anka and Molly: they normally accompany me in a peaceful fashion, stopping endlessly to investigate interesting smells. If, however, we chance to encounter a cat, a squirrel, or, worse still, a sheep, they are transformed into hunters and, wrenching their leads from my anxious grip, they are off and away, lead handles thundering down the road. Last year, just before Christmas, we encountered a cat outside the Lord Mayor's official residence. Before I knew it, I was flat on my face on the cobblestones with two broken teeth and the dogs were off down the road. I should explain that chows are not to be confused with Pomeranians, and Molly and Anka's combined weight is sixty-three kilos, exactly equal to mine. So I am no match for them when the blood lust is upon them.

The real joy of these creatures, of course, is that they love me as much as I love them. Around the house they are a quiet presence but if I have been away their welcome is quite overwhelming. I have been away lecturing several times this year – in Dublin, Kuala Lumpur and Australia – as well as my summer visit to Maine. I hate leaving the dogs but have a wonderful team of friends who will walk and feed them and, if necessary, dog-sit in my flat.

Living at such close proximity with these only partially domesticated creatures is a constant fascination to me as I observe their behaviour and marvel that I share their space and life. I am entranced, too, by many of the television wildlife programmes, especially the ones exploring the behaviour of the big cats. We are privileged to live in an era in which animal photography is so sophisticated that we can now see into a creature's burrow or nest and watch it give birth and tend its young. I am reminded of the passage in Job where Yahweh speaks from the heart of the tempest:

> Do you know how mountain goats give birth,
> or have you ever watched the hinds in labour?
> How many months do they carry their young?
> At what time do they give birth? (Job 39:1–2)

David Attenborough, veteran producer of hundreds of wonderful nature films, probably *does* know how the mountain goats give birth, but there are still endless areas of undiscovered animal behaviour. These programmes are important to me because they help me cultivate my sense of wonder in God and the universe. Occasionally I meet people who proudly declare that they don't own a television but I believe them to be the poorer for it. I get so much enjoyment from my TV, watching not only the nature but also travel and history programmes. My favourites, however, I have to admit are the medical and police dramas and my friends always think twice before telephoning me after eight o'clock in the evening!

While I watch television, I knit baby blankets, and sweaters for my sister and my friends. I love the gentle movement of the needles and rejoice in the colour and texture of the yarn. My knitting hero is Kaffe Fassett, a Californian artist who changed British knitting for ever, creating his garments like a painting with beautiful bright or subtle colours, mixing yarn types with a freedom which would have shocked the more conservative. I always thought that when I retired I would take up painting in oils but, like my mother before me, I am more at home with fabric and yarn.

All the women in my family have a passion for, and a way with, colour. We love oriental rugs and blue and white china, along with various *objets d'art* purchased while abroad. On my mantelpiece I have a terracotta mother and child from Shanghai, a wooden horse and warrior from Burma, purchased this year in Bangkok, and a lovely glazed Chinese horse, a modern facsimile of the fabulous Tang dynasty horses which cost hundreds of pounds. My heart still lusts after a thousand-year-old large terracotta chow which I saw in a very exclusive shop in Bangkok on my way back from Australia this year. I did, however, find a small jade chow in Melbourne and he has pride of place next to a (probably fake) jade horse purchased from an old, old woman on the banks of the Yangtze Kiang River a few years back.

In August 2005 I was encouraged to reflect more seriously on the family genes and their pattern of inheritance when I was invited to be honorary head of the Cassidy clan worldwide for the next three years. On Saturday 6 August I was crowned, or rather inaugurated, as head of the clan at a ceremony on Devenish Island in County Fermanagh, an ancient monastic settlement where there are a number of Cassidy graves. I was welcomed as 'An Caisideach', 'The Cassidy', by clan members from Ireland, the USA, England and Australia, and handed a hazel rod mounted with the silver hand of Nuada and a number of documents concerning Devenish Island and the Cassidys. These symbolic articles were inspired by the Cassidys' prominence in the fields of literature, medicine and religion in Fermanagh for over a thousand years. At the close of the ceremony the group sang a hymn, Moelisa Dixit, composed by St Molaise, the founding abbot of Devenish Monastery in the sixth century. It is a simple hymn inviting the Holy Spirit to come to us, to be in us and with us.

There was another poem, even older than Moelisa Dixit, which produced in me shivers of delight at the stunning imagery used to evoke the Divine. This poem, known as 'The Song of Amergin', is said to be the first poem uttered in Ireland.

> I am the Wind that blows across the Sea;
> I am the Wave of the Ocean;
> I am the Murmur of the Billows;
> I am the Bull of the Seven Combats;
> I am the Vulture on the Rock;
> I am a Ray of the Sun;
> I am the Fairest of Flowers;
> I am a Wild Boar in Valour;
> I am a Salmon in the Pool;
> I am a Lake on the Plain;
> I am the Skill of the Craftsman;
> I am a Word of Science;
> I am the Spear-point that gives Battle;
> I am the God who creates in the head of man the Fire of
>   Thought;
> Who is it Enlightens the Assembly upon the mountain, if not I?
> Who tells the ages of the moon, if not I?
> Who shows the place where the sun goes to rest, if not I?
> Who calls the cattle from the House of Tethra?
> On whom do the cattle of Tethra smile?
> Who is the God that fashions enchantments – the enchantment
>   of battle and the wind of change?
>
> From 'Leabhar Gabhala'

As I transcribe this verse I am conscious of my Celtic blood and of how many ways there are to encounter and evoke the Divine. Some might see this as pagan nature worship, but I don't. This thrills my soul in the way that Gregorian chant does, or the majestic tolling of the big bell for the grand silence at Ampleforth Abbey. The God in whom I believe is everywhere: in the Eucharist, in my garden, in the clients with whom I work and in my dogs.

He or she has led me a merry dance into the torture chamber and out, into the convent and out, and then through twenty years of the most satisfying work a woman could wish for. Now I have emerged into a sunlit meadow and I feel God's love like the sun on my back. I have no idea what joy or suffering the future may bring but I am ready for either. I end with a prayer from my convent school days which I made very much my own in prison:

> Grant that I may love thee always,
> then do with me what thou wilt.

NOTES
1. Ann Lewin, *Candles and Kingfishers: Reflections on the Journey* (Foundery Press, 1997), p. 21.
2. In Philip Larkin, *High Windows* (Faber and Faber, 1979).